Applied Anatomy for
Clinical Procedures
at a Glance

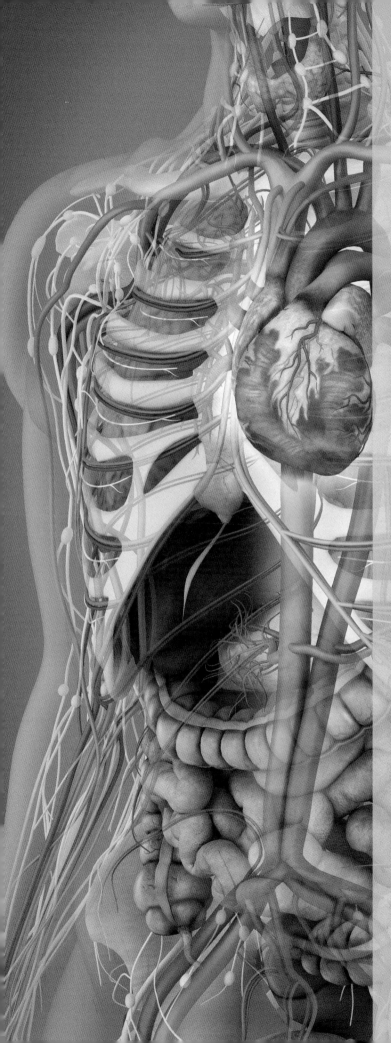

Applied Anatomy for Clinical Procedures at a Glance

Jane Sturgess

Francesca Crawley

Ramez Kirollos

Kirsty Cattle

WILEY Blackwell

This edition first published 2021
© 2021 John Wiley & Sons Ltd.

The right of Jane Sturgess, Francesca Crawley, Ramez Kirollos, and Kirsty Cattle to be identified as the author(s) of this work has been asserted in accordance with law.

Registered Office(s)
John Wiley & Sons, Inc., 111 River Street, Hoboken, NJ 07030, USA
John Wiley & Sons Ltd, The Atrium, Southern Gate, Chichester, West Sussex, PO19 8SQ, UK

Editorial Office
111 River Street, Hoboken, NJ 07030, USA

For details of our global editorial offices, customer services, and more information about Wiley products visit us at www.wiley.com.

Wiley also publishes its books in a variety of electronic formats and by print-on-demand. Some content that appears in standard print versions of this book may not be available in other formats.

Library of Congress Cataloging-in-Publication Data

Names: Sturgess, Jane, author. | Crawley, Francesca, author. | Kirollos,
    Ramez, author. | Cattle, Kirsty, author.
Title: Applied anatomy for clinical procedures at a glance / Jane Sturgess,
    Francesca Crawley, Ramez Kirollos, Kirsty Cattle.
Other titles: At a glance series (Oxford, England)
Description: Hoboken, NJ : Wiley-Blackwell 2021. | Series: At a glance
    series | Includes bibliographical references and index.
Identifiers: LCCN 2020015329 (print) | LCCN 2020015330 (ebook) | ISBN
    9781119054580 (paperback) | ISBN 9781119054610 (adobe pdf) | ISBN
    9781119054641 (epub)
Subjects: MESH: Surgical Procedures, Operative | Diagnostic Techniques and
    Procedures | Clinical Medicine–methods | Anatomy | Handbook
Classification: LCC RD37 (print) | LCC RD37 (ebook) | NLM WO 39 | DDC
    617–dc23
LC record available at https://lccn.loc.gov/2020015329
LC ebook record available at https://lccn.loc.gov/2020015330

Cover Design: Wiley
Cover Image: © Stocktrek Images/Getty Images

Set in 9.5/11.5pt Minion Pro by SPi Global, Pondicherry, India
Printed and bound in Singapore by Markono Print Media Pte Ltd

10 9 8 7 6 5 4 3 2 1

Contents

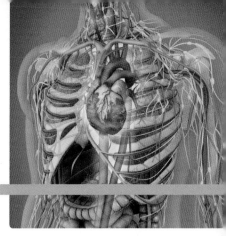

Contributors

Kirsty Cattle
East of England Deanery
Cambridge, UK

Charles Crawley
Addenbrooke's Hospital
Cambridge University Hospitals NHS Trust
Cambridge, UK

Francesca Crawley
West Suffolk Hospital
Bury St Edmunds, UK

Olivia Kenyon
East of England Deanery
Cambridge, UK

Ramez Kirollos
Addenbrooke's Hospital
Cambridge University Hospitals NHS Trust
Cambridge, UK

Sherif Kirollos
Addenbrooke's Hospital
Cambridge University Hospitals NHS Trust
Cambridge, UK

Jane Sturgess
West Suffolk Hospital
Bury St Edmunds, UK

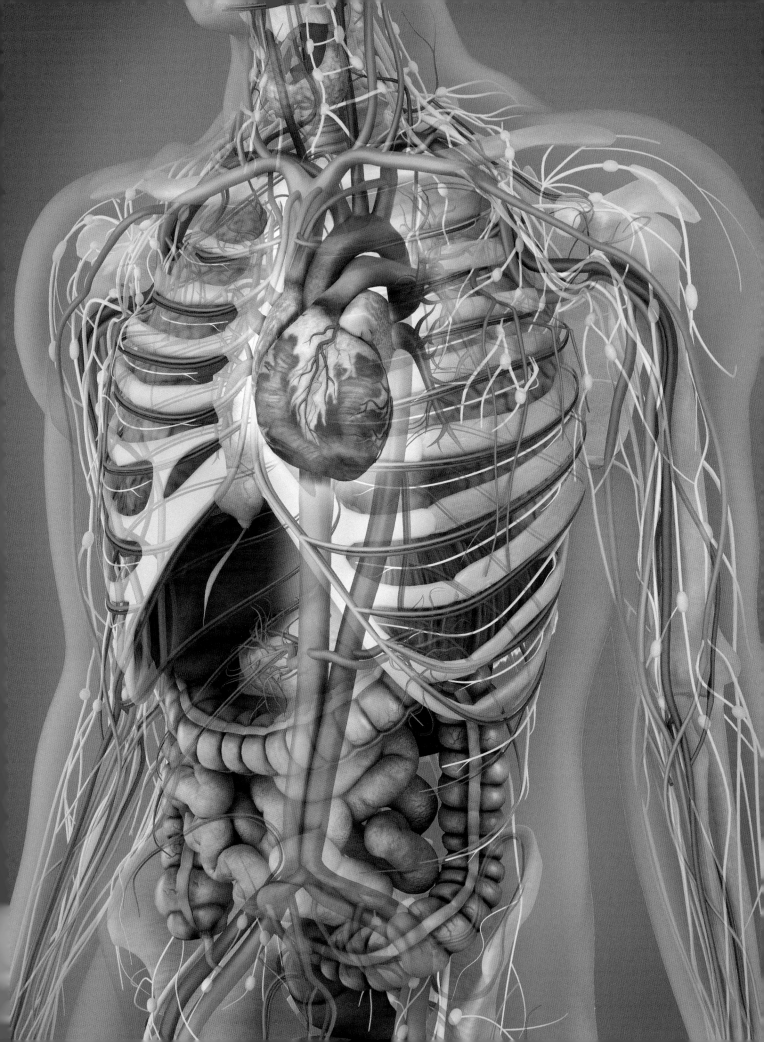

Scrubbing up

Sherif Kirollos and Ramez Kirollos

Figure 1.1 Equipment.

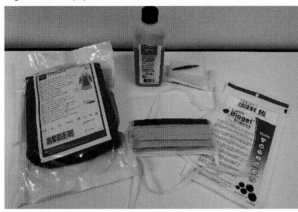

Figure 1.2 Before scrubbing, don hat, mask, eye protection.

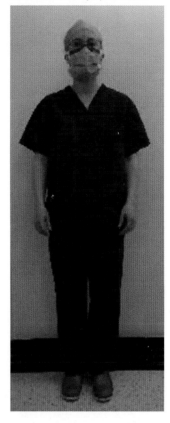

Figure 1.3 Recommended handwashing technique.

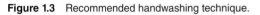

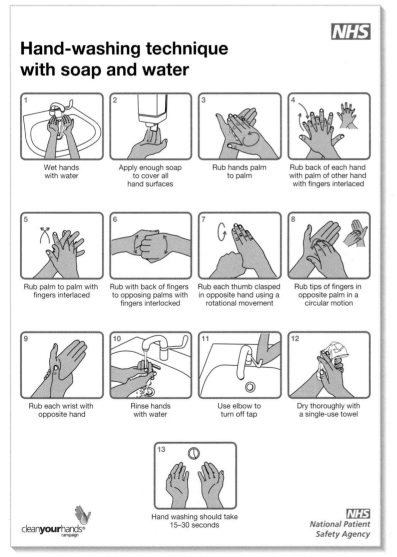

NHS

Hand-washing technique with soap and water

1. Wet hands with water
2. Apply enough soap to cover all hand surfaces
3. Rub hands palm to palm
4. Rub back of each hand with palm of other hand with fingers interlaced
5. Rub palm to palm with fingers interlaced
6. Rub with back of fingers to opposing palms with fingers interlocked
7. Rub each thumb clasped in opposite hand using a rotational movement
8. Rub tips of fingers in opposite palm in a circular motion
9. Rub each wrist with opposite hand
10. Rinse hands with water
11. Use elbow to turn off tap
12. Dry thoroughly with a single-use towel
13. Hand washing should take 15–30 seconds

clean**your**hands®
campaign

NHS
National Patient Safety Agency

Applied Anatomy for Clinical Procedures at a Glance, First Edition. Jane Sturgess, Francesca Crawley, Ramez Kirollos, and Kirsty Cattle.
© 2021 John Wiley & Sons Ltd. Published 2021 by John Wiley & Sons Ltd.

Figure 1.4 Procedure. (a) Wash hands and arms three times (b) rinsing from fingertips to elbows between each wash. (c) Dry skin thoroughly, from hands down to elbows. (d) Don gown and gloves touching only the inside of each.

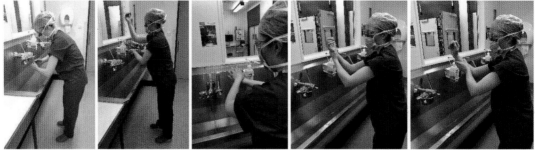

(a)

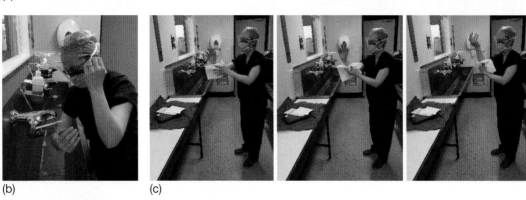

(b)   (c)

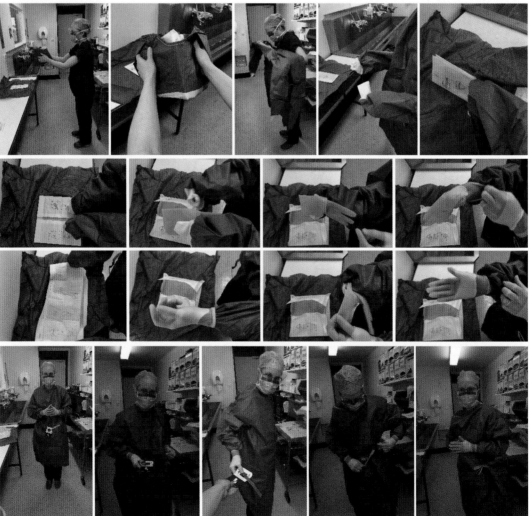

(d)

Equipment (Figure 1.1)

- Antiseptic solution [either povidone iodine (Betadine) or chlorhexidine]
- Gown
- Gloves
- Face mask
- Nail brush

Antiseptic solutions

The common antiseptics used for scrubbing are povidone iodine (Betadine) and chlorhexidine. These are applied to the skin and have a bactericidal or bacteriostatic effect, but complete asepsis (sterility) is not achieved.

Chlorhexidine: This is a cationic polybiguanide which achieves both a bacteriostatic and bactericidal effect depending on its concentration, through the release of charged cations which bind to and disrupt the bacterial cell wall. This solution is effective against a broad range of organisms, including gram-positive and gram-negative organisms, aerobes, anaerobes, and yeasts.

Povidone iodine: This is a solution containing a combination of iodine and polyvinylpyrrolidone (PVP). A bactericidal effect is achieved through the molecular iodine, and PVP acts as an iodophor to prevent irritation and toxicity to the tissue by keeping the free iodine concentration low. The solution acts against gram-positive and gram-negative bacteria, bacterial spores, viruses, protozoa, and fungi.

Procedure (Figure 1.4)

1. The hair is first covered by a hat and a mask is worn. Depending on the procedure protective eye goggles may be used. For specific procedures, a hooded surgical gown can be used (Figure 1.2).

2. For the first scrubbing in of the day, handwashing should last for 5 minutes, and subsequent handwashing should allow 3 minutes each, following the recommended handwashing procedure (Figure 1.3).

3. Any breach of the procedure requires recommencing of the cycle.

4. Antiseptic washing must cover all aspects of the skin of the hands and forearms, extending to the elbows. Particular attention should be paid to the interdigital spaces and under the nails. A brush may be used to apply the antiseptic solution to the skin under the nails but is best avoided elsewhere to avoid causing superficial skin abrasions with more vigorous scrubbing as that would expose underlying cutaneous bacteria.

5. During handwashing, ensure that hands and forearms remain elevated, allowing the water to drip from the elbow to avoid contamination as a result of water running from unsterile regions to areas already cleaned. Shaking should also be avoided for the same reason.

6. Throughout the handwashing cycles, ensure enough time is allowed for contact of the antiseptic with the skin before running it under water.

7. The skin is then dried with sterile towels while avoiding contact with unsterile regions (Figure 1.4c).

8. As contact with non-sterile surroundings is prevented, the gown is then delivered from its sterile wrapping and donned (Figure 1.4d).

9. The arms and hands are kept within the sleeves until gloves are worn without touching their outer surface. This can be achieved by initially avoiding protruding the fingers through the gown sleeves. Alternatively, the surgeon is helped by an assistant or a scrub nurse holding open each pair of gloves.

2 Setting up a sterile field and draping the patient

Sherif Kirollos and Ramez Kirollos

Figure 2.1 Equipment.

Figure 2.2 Apply the antiseptic to the operating field in a radial or concentric movement, away from the operating site.

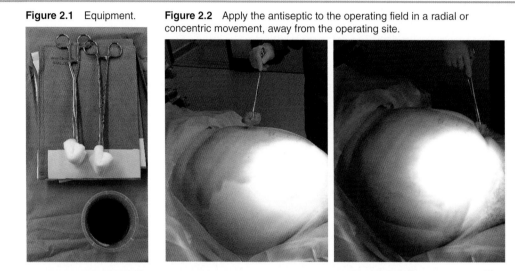

Figure 2.3 Cover the edges of the operating field with sterile drapes, adhering them to sterilised skin.

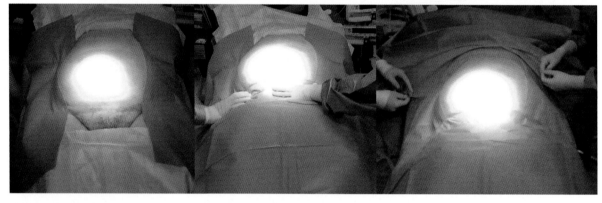

Figure 2.4 Use of an antiseptic impregnated incise drape reduces surgical site infection.

Figure 2.5 Use sterile drapes to cover an operating trolley on which operating instruments and equipment will be placed.

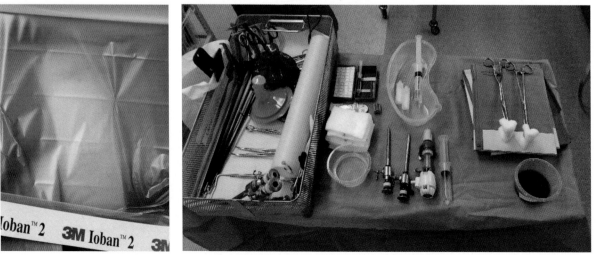

A sterile field includes the exposed area of the patient to be operated upon or the region through which the trajectory of the procedure crosses. The sterile field also involves the area where the instruments and equipment used for the procedure are placed.

Equipment (Figure 2.1)

- Antiseptics (see Chapter 1, Scrubbing up)
- Sponge holder forceps
- Drapes and plastic adhesive incise drape
- Towel holders
- Light handle
- Masks
- Sterile gloves
- Gown

Procedure

1. Hair shaving requires a balanced view as shaving the skin area prior to surgery potentially exposes cutaneous and hair follicle bacteria; however, excessive hair in the operating field may hinder sealing of the operating field with adhesive drapes. If no or minimal shaving is adopted, then ensure application of antiseptic (shampoo) to a wider area.
2. Sterile sponge holder forceps with sterile swabs are immersed in an antiseptic solution which is applied to the skin or mucous membrane which is to be sterilised. A prior check regarding allergies to the antiseptic should be completed.
3. Applying the antiseptic solution to the operating field is recommended to be in a radial or concentric movement away from the operative site to avoid contamination from a non-sterile region. This applies particularly in areas proximal to potentially contaminated areas such as the anal orifice or the umbilicus (Figure 2.2).
4. Sterile drapes and towels are used to cover the margins of the exposed and cleaned patient's skin (Figure 2.3).
5. The skin area to be draped should be cleaned with a generous margin to achieve adequate exposure. This may include adjacent anatomical landmarks used for orientation, for example when operating on the face.
6. The drapes are fixed with an overlying plastic adhesive incise drape to prevent contamination from skin organisms. Antiseptic impregnated incise drapes are recommended to decrease surgical infection (Figure 2.4).
7. The surface of the operating trolley on which the instruments and equipment are to be placed is covered with sterile towels (Figure 2.5). Drapes can also be used to 'shield' the sterile area. It is important to maintain the sterility of the surface of the instrument trolleys and the equipment until the end of the procedure.
8. At the end of the surgical procedure, disposable sharp objects and contaminated material should be disposed of in the appropriate containers.

Top tips

- The antiseptic has its bactericidal effect by drying. Using a smaller volume of antiseptic and allowing it to dry will have a better sterilising effect than using larger volumes of antiseptic.

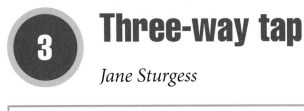

3 Three-way tap

Jane Sturgess

Figure 3.1 Three-way tap. Note the arrows on the limbs to indicate flow of fluid/air.

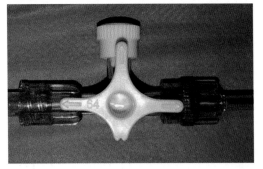

Figure 3.2 Equipment. Three-way taps come individually or incorporated with extension tubing.

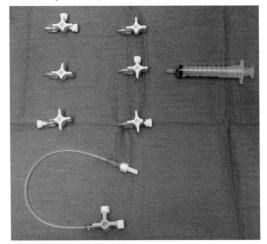

Figure 3.3 Different possible positions of a three-way tap and combinations of equipment: (a) open to infusion and cannula; (b) open to infusion, air, and cannula; (c) as per b but capped off to air; (d) used for aspirating from cannula or injecting intravenously; (e) open to infusion, syringe, and cannula; (f) open to infusion and syringe – useful for aspirating fluid to then give bolus by turning three-way tap round to position d; (g) used for giving two infusions simultaneously; (h) off to all ports.

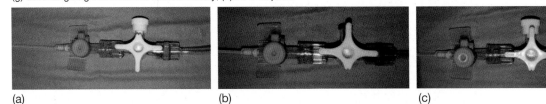

(a)

(b)

(c)

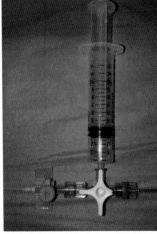

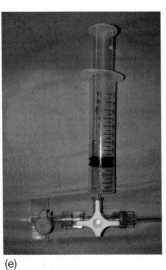

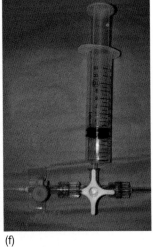

(d)

(e)

(f)

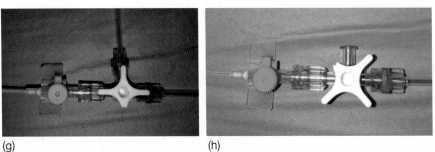

(g)

(h)

Applied Anatomy for Clinical Procedures at a Glance, First Edition. Jane Sturgess, Francesca Crawley, Ramez Kirollos, and Kirsty Cattle.
© 2021 John Wiley & Sons Ltd. Published 2021 by John Wiley & Sons Ltd.

Description of the three-way tap

The three-way tap is shaped like a T, and when examined closely you can see each 'arm' of the 'T' has a small arrow or line on it (Figure 3.1). The arrow indicates that flow can happen through it, as long as the arrow is pointing at something that permits flow – like a fluid line, a vein, or air.

Another way to look at the three-way tap is to imagine it like a road traffic roundabout with three exits. Flow can happen only when there is an exit attached to an open secondary route (giving line, fluid circuit, air). If the exit has a bung on it imagine it like a roadblock: flow does not occur.

The top of the 'T' with no arm (and no arrow), or the aspect of the 'roundabout' with no exit, stops flow and acts as an off switch.

It may come individually or be incorporated with extension tubing (Figure 3.2).

Potential uses of the three-way tap (Figure 3.3)

1. To aspirate fluid from a fluid giving set
2. To aspirate fluid from a drain (e.g. ascitic drain, pleural drain)
3. To aspirate blood from invasive lines (e.g. central venous pressure [CVP] or arterial line)
4. To aspirate air from a fluid giving set
5. To aspirate air from a drain (examples as 2)
6. To permit intermittent pressure measurements with a manometer in a fluid system (e.g. cerebrospinal fluid [CSF] pressure, invasive blood pressure, intra-abdominal pressure)
7. To inject drugs into a fluid-filled system (e.g. intravenous fluid giving set, CSF injection, epidural catheter, external ventricular drain)
8. To inject drugs, treatments into other spaces (e.g. pleurodesis)
9. To permit the infusion of more than one fluid or drug at the same time via the same cannula

Safe use of a three-way tap

The three-way tap acts as an interface between the patient and the therapy; either as a middle point between lines into or drains from the patient, and a giving/monitoring set, or a drain collection device.

Look at the tap, identify the arms, and decide which way to turn it before going ahead with the procedure. It is also worth planning to use a bung if you need to stop flow through one of the arms (even if for a short time or as a temporary measure). Whilst planning how to turn the taps during the procedure, you should also decide how you need to leave the tap when the procedure is finished; should flow be permitted to continue, or does it need to be stopped.

If an arm of the T, or a road exit is pointing to an open exit with no device or bung attached it is 'open to air'. This presents a significant risk of either (i) air entering the patient and causing a serious complication, for example, air embolus, pneumothorax, pneumocephalus OR (ii) fluid leaving the patient in an unplanned and/or uncontrolled manner, for example, bleeding, fast and excessive loss of CSF, ascites, or pleural fluid.

It is important to use a clean technique when using or manipulating the three-way tap for infection control to protect the patient and to avoid cross-contamination of any samples taken.

After the procedure

Make sure there are no arms left open to air.

When deciding how to leave the tap at the end of a procedure it is worth thinking about what measure you will use to determine whether and when to change your plan – this measure may be determined by time, by patient's symptoms (increasing breathlessness), by pressure measurement (CSF pressure greater than 15 cmH$_2$O), by volume of fluid in the drain etc.

Your first plan may be to permit flow or to stop flow.

Anatomical pitfalls

1. If the fluid/air you hope to drain is at high pressure or high volume it will automatically flow to the outside – take care if this is unplanned, or you wish to drain only a predetermined amount (e.g. pleural effusion, CSF, ascites). Be prepared to replace large fluid losses with the appropriate intravenous replacement fluid (blood, albumin, crystalloid).
2. If the fluid/air you hope to drain is at low pressure (negative intrapleural pressure on inspiration, or central vein with three-way tap system above the level of the heart) or low volume, fluid may flow into the patient inadvertently causing complications such as pneumothorax or air embolism – take care.
3. Using a syringe to aspirate a low volume, low pressure system can collapse the tissues if too great a negative pressure is applied. This can either make the drain or line fail or give a false negative result to your aspiration, leading to unnecessary repeated tests (with associated risks) or a false diagnostic conclusion (with associated risks, and delay in diagnosis).

Top tips

1. Look at the tap and plan how to turn it before you start – which ways do you need fluid/air to flow and at what time points of the procedure?
2. Plan how to stop flow – you can either turn the tap so that the top of the T with no arm faces the direction you want to stop flow from (usually the patient); you can put a bung onto the Luer lock that has an arm with an arrow pointing towards it; or you can quarter turn the tap so that none of the arms point towards a line – it will lie at an angle to the giving system.
3. If aspirating low volume or low pressure fluid consider using a small syringe in the first instance and be prepared with a choice of larger syringes. It is easy to switch to a larger syringe during the procedure if the fluid/air flows easily.

4 Common equipment for core clinical procedures

Jane Sturgess

Figure 4.1 Image to show the possible types of needle tip and position of the lumen. Most needles for procedures and all cannulas have a quincke (or cutting) tip. Sprotte and Whitacre tips are found on spinal needles.

Common tip design for spinal needles

Quincke

Whitacre

Sprotte

Figure 4.2 Butterfly needles. Note the needle length and injection port (white hub) are standard across the sizes. The diameter of the needle and tubing, the colour and design of the 'wings' differ. The green butterfly has a vacutainer attachment at the white hub.

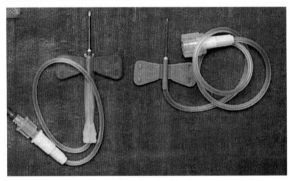

Figure 4.3 Spinal needles. Note the difference in needle diameter for each colour.

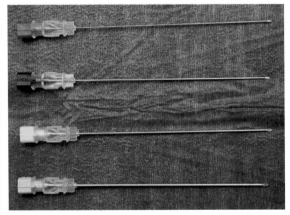

Figure 4.4 Cannulas. Note the difference in needle diameter and length for each colour.

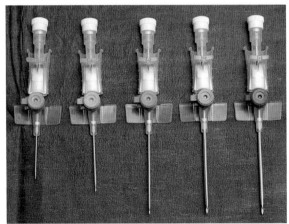

Figure 4.5 Syringes. Note the different tips of the 60 mL syringes. From left to right - NG aspiration/injection, Luer tip, Luer-Lok for use with infusion tubing, bladder tip.

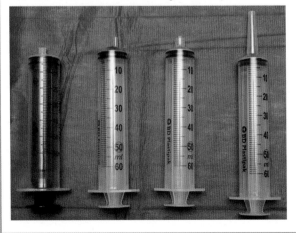

Figure 4.6 Urinary catheters. From top to bottom 3 way, 2 way, Curved or Coude tip, soft 2 way.

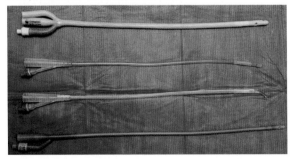

Applied Anatomy for Clinical Procedures at a Glance, First Edition. Jane Sturgess, Francesca Crawley, Ramez Kirollos, and Kirsty Cattle.
© 2021 John Wiley & Sons Ltd. Published 2021 by John Wiley & Sons Ltd.

Figure 4.7   Urinary catheter bags. The most commonly used bag in hospital has the urometer (the large plastic reservoir), permitting accurate urine hourly output measurements.

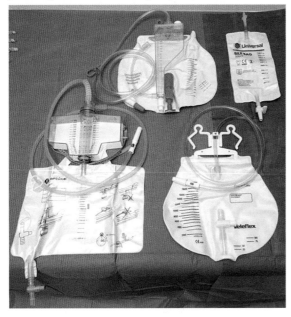

Figure 4.8   Commonly used blood bottles.

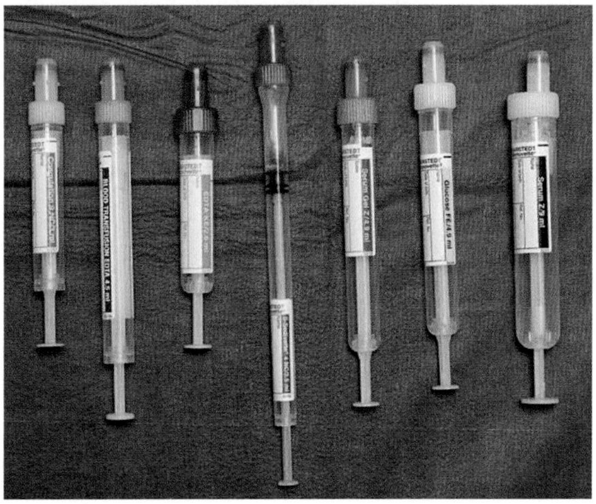

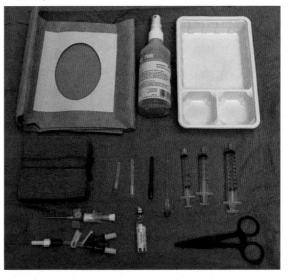

Figure 4.9   Blood culture bottles.

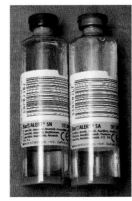

Figure 4.10   Sample pots. The white capped pot is suitable to collect most samples for core procedures.

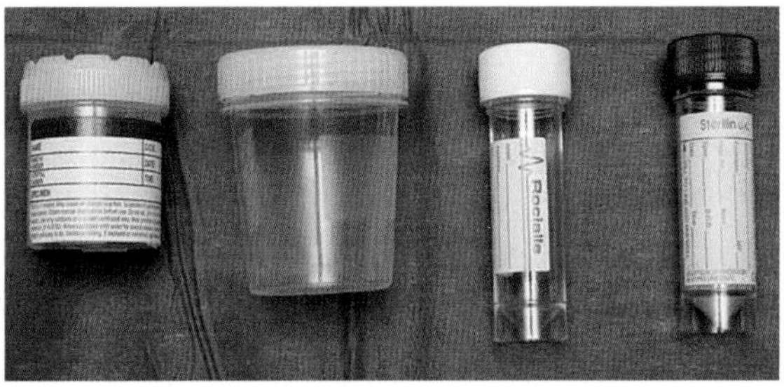

Figure 4.11   Simple dressing pack, often used for small procedures.

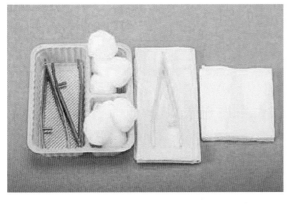

Figure 4.12   Large sterile pack, for central lines and more invasive procedures.

Needles

These can be sharp (for procedures) or blunt (for drawing up), hollow or not (suture needles), and have the lumen at the end of the needle or at the side (Figure 4.1).

Hollow needles

	Size	Length	Common Use
Orange	25 G	16 mm	To raise a skin wheal with local anaesthetic
Blue	23 G	30 mm	Deeper tissue infiltration with local anaesthetic or to locate the depth of fluid-filled cavities (e.g. pleural space). To take arterial blood gases
Green	21 G	40 mm	As for Blue, but also to take blood from peripheral or iliac vein
White	19 G	50 mm	
Red (Blunt)	18 G	40 mm	Draw up drugs
Red filter	18 G	40 mm	Draw up drugs when particulate matter (glass fragments from vial, microbes) MUST be avoided (e.g. intrathecal injection of drug)

G = gauge

Butterflies

All come with 300 mm length tubing, a universal port at the end, and a bung which may need changing to a bionector for safety and infection control (Figure 4.2).

	Size	Diameter
Ivory	19 G	1.2 mm
Green	21 G	0.8 mm
Blue	23 G	0.6 mm
Orange	25 G	0.5 mm

Spinal needles (Figure 4.3)

	Size	Tip	Lumen	Common Use
Orange	25 G	Pencil Point	Side	Intrathecal drug delivery. Comes with introducer needle
Black (standard)	22 G	Quincke	End	Lumbar puncture. (90 mm)
Black (long)	22 G	Quincke	End	Lumbar puncture in the obese (127 mm)
Yellow	20 G	Quincke	End	
Pink	18 G	Quincke	End	

Cannulas (Figure 4.4)

The flow rate that can be achieved through a cannula depends on its brand, the height of the fluid bag above the cannula site, and whether a pressure bag is applied. Simple physics dictates that the wider the lumen of the cannula and the greater the pressure gradient, the faster the flow.

	Size	Length*	Flow*	Common Use
Yellow	25 G	19 mm	24 mL/min	Paediatrics
Blue	22 G	25 mm	42 mL/min	Difficult access or simple medication
Pink	20 G	32 mm	67 mL/min	Fluids and medication
Green	18 G	45 mm	103 mL/min	Blood transfusion
Grey	16 G	45 mm	236 mL/min	Resuscitation
Orange	14 G	45 mm	330 mL/min	Rapid resuscitation

*Flows based on BD™ Venflon Pro Safety without a pressure bag.

Syringes (Figure 4.5)

Syringes with Luer and Luer-Lok™ tips can be attached to needles, three-way taps, and bionector connections. For safety reasons special tips have been designed to attach to nasogastric (NG) tubes, and newer separate tips are being designed and may become available for intrathecal or epidural drug delivery systems.

NB. When aspirating fluid be mindful that forceful displacement of the plunger on smaller syringes can create a large negative pressure at the tip of the syringe (Pressure = force/area) and collapse veins or fluid filled cavities. Choose the appropriate syringe according to volume of fluid present and withdraw the plunger slowly and steadily.

	Tip	Common Use
1 mL	Luer	Insulin (there are specific insulin syringes that MUST be used), or for low dose drugs where accuracy is crucial
2 mL	Luer	Local anaesthesia (LA) for arterial blood gases, or as a reservoir when adjusting difficult cannulas etc
5 mL	Luer	LA for field anaesthesia
10 mL	Luer	Taking blood, some drug dilutions, some needle aspirates
20 mL	Luer	Aspiration of large volumes of fluid, for example, pleural effusion, knee effusion, or for blood cultures
50 mL	Luer	Aspiration of very large fluid volumes.
Bladder syringe	Catheter	To flush a blocked catheter, or to aspirate urine.
NG syringe	NG specific	To give drugs or water, or to remove gastric secretions

Sampling devices

Urinary catheters (Figure 4.6)

Available in a number of sizes, measured in French (Fr) gauge. The higher the Fr number, the larger the catheter (opposite to intravenous cannulae where a larger number indicates a smaller diameter lumen). The Foley and coude can be connected to simple or hourly drainage bags.

Straight, single use	Single lumen	Small 1.25 cm opening	Often used for self-catheterisation
2-way Foley	Inflatable balloon near the tip		Retention catheters – most commonly used in hospital
3-way Foley	Inflatable balloon near the tip	Variety of sizes	Used for bladder irrigation following prostate or bladder surgery
Curved or coude	Curved tip		Useful in patients with prostatic hypertrophy

Catheter bags (Figure 4.7)

These can be provided as a simple collection system for patients with a urinary catheter (but not on strict fluid balance observations) or with an urometer to permit hourly measurements. All are supplied sterile with a non-return valve to prevent ascending infection.

Commonly used blood bottles (Figures 4.8 and 4.9)

	Volume	Contains	Tests
Purple	>1 mL (4 mL)	EDTA	FBC, Blood film, PTH, ESR, HbA1c
Pink	6 mL	EDTA	G&S, cross-match, direct Coombs
Blue	2.7 mL	Sodium citrate	Coagulation, INR, D-dimer, APTT, Factor-Xa
Yellow/Gold	>1 mL (5 mL)	Silica particles	U&E, Creatinine, most biochemistry
Grey	2 mL	Sodium fluoride, potassium oxalate	Glucose, lactate
Red	6 mL	Silica particles	Hormones, toxicology, serology
Dark Green		Heparin	Insulin, renin, aldosterone
Black			ESR (paediatrics)
Blood Culture	8–10 mL per bottle	Culture medium	Blue lid – aerobic culture, Purple lid – anaerobic culture

APTT = activated partial thromboplastin time; ESR = erythrocyte sedimentation rate; FBC = full blood count; G&S = group & screen; INR = International Normalised Ratio; PTH = parathyroid hormone; U&E = urea and electrolytes.

Sample pots (Figure 4.10)

These typically are preservative free with a white screw cap top and are available in a number of sizes. The most commonly used is a 30 mL pot, which is suitable for cerebrospinal fluid, sputum, urine.

Sterile procedure packs (Figures 4.11 and 4.12)

These will often be custom made for the hospital/GP practice you are working in. A key tip is 'less is more'. The simplest pack you use should be wrapped in a sterile towel that forms the basis of your sterile working area and contains a small pot for cleaning fluid and some gauze or cotton wool. You (or an assistant) can open needles, syringes, sutures, and sample pots onto the sterile area. The key consideration is 'how large does my sterile field need to be?'; this will guide your choice of pack.

5 Local anaesthetic infiltration

Sherif Kirollos and Ramez Kirollos

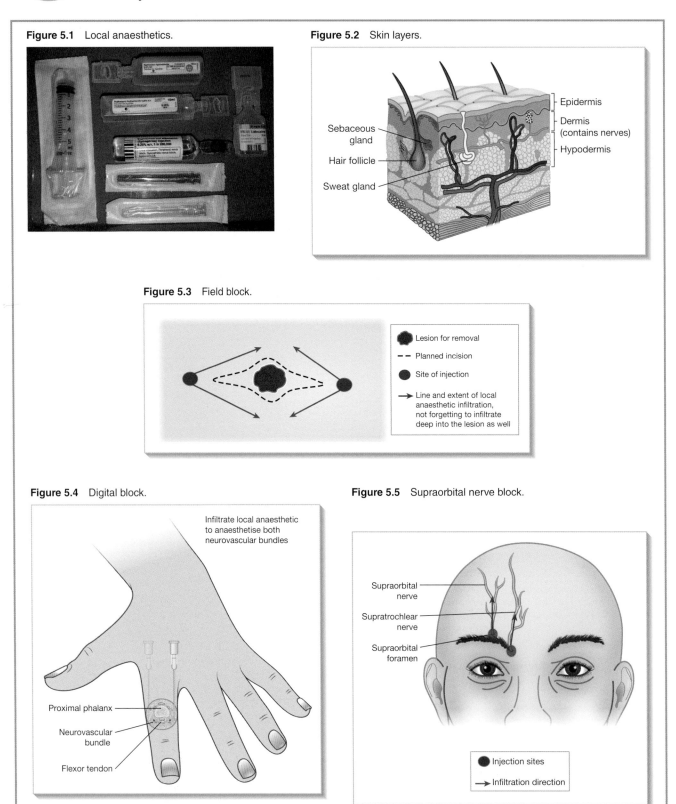

Figure 5.1   Local anaesthetics.

Figure 5.2   Skin layers.

Epidermis

Dermis (contains nerves)

Hypodermis

Sebaceous gland

Hair follicle

Sweat gland

Figure 5.3   Field block.

Lesion for removal

Planned incision

Site of injection

Line and extent of local anaesthetic infiltration, not forgetting to infiltrate deep into the lesion as well

Figure 5.4   Digital block.

Infiltrate local anaesthetic to anaesthetise both neurovascular bundles

Proximal phalanx

Neurovascular bundle

Flexor tendon

Figure 5.5   Supraorbital nerve block.

Supraorbital nerve

Supratrochlear nerve

Supraorbital foramen

Injection sites

Infiltration direction

Applied Anatomy for Clinical Procedures at a Glance, First Edition. Jane Sturgess, Francesca Crawley, Ramez Kirollos, and Kirsty Cattle.
© 2021 John Wiley & Sons Ltd. Published 2021 by John Wiley & Sons Ltd.

Classes of local anaesthetics (Figure 5.1)

Local anaesthetics generally fall into one of two classes: aminoamide (such as lidocaine and bupivacaine) or aminoester (procaine, tetracaine, and chloroprocaine). Lidocaine is a commonly used local anaesthetic, typically provided in 1% or 2% concentrations.

Mechanism of action

Non-ionised local anaesthetics cross the lipid bilayer of the cell where they become ionised. The ionised form reversibly binds to voltage-gated sodium channels. This inhibits the function of nerve endings by preventing the inward current of sodium, thereby preventing the rapid depolarisation of nerve cells and hence preventing an action potential. As they show a greater affinity for channels in their open and inactivated states, their effect is greatest on frequently depolarising nerve cells.

Dose

The dose of lidocaine is 7 mg/kg when combined with adrenaline (3–5 mg/kg without adrenaline). The doses for other agents differ; for example, bupivacaine is used at almost half the dose of lidocaine.

When calculating the dose, considerations should be given to the presence of adrenaline in the preparation, the strength of the preparation, dilution, and body weight. The maximum dose may be modified where there is a history of heart disease to avoid toxicity.

As an example, a 1% lidocaine preparation contains 10 mg/mL of lidocaine. Therefore to administer this to a 70 kg patient in the recommended dose of 4 mg/kg, the maximum volume this patient can receive is 280 mg or 28 mL of lidocaine (1%).

Lidocaine has an onset of approximately 2 to 5 mins, with a lasting effect of up to 2 hours, whereas bupivacaine takes effect after 20–30 mins but has a longer acting effect of up to 4 hours. The two can be used in combination to take advantage of both their properties.

The vasoconstrictive effect of adrenaline reduces the rate at which the anaesthetic is removed from the circulation and therefore prolongs the analgesic effect.

Side effects

1. Central nervous system neurotoxicity: Initial symptoms and signs may include tinnitus, perioral numbness, diplopia, nystagmus, slurred speech, and metallic taste. Higher doses may progress to the development of irritability, fine tremors, and even seizures or respiratory arrest.

2. Cardiac: As local anaesthetics are also classified as antiarrhythmic drugs, such as lidocaine as a class 1b antiarrhythmic, they have the effect of reducing the rate of cardiac muscle depolarisation. As the concentration of the anesthetic agent is increased, the velocity of cardiac action potential is decreased. Therefore, at toxic doses, this will have a greater negative inotropic effect and may lead to bradycardia, fibrillation, or asystole. Hypotension may also occur due to their direct vasodilatory effect on peripheral arteriolar smooth muscles.

3. Respiratory: Toxic doses may depress respiration.

4. Systemic: Hypersensitivity reactions are extremely rare but are important to recognise. They may be the result of either a type I or type IV reaction.

Technique

1. Clean the site with antiseptic.
2. Wipe the top of the bottle with an alcohol wipe.
3. Using a wide bore needle and syringe, draw up the appropriate volume of anaesthetic and remove any air left in the syringe while keeping it upright.
4. Replace the wide bore needle with a smaller gauge needle (such as a 25 gauge needle).
5. Making sure the bevel of the needle is facing up, insert the needle into the site and aspirate to ensure there has been no entry into a blood vessel. Initially inject a small amount superficially which raises a dermal 'bleb', then advance as deep as needed (see Figure 5.2). Ensure to aspirate first and then inject increasing volumes of anaesthetic as the needle is withdrawn to cover the area as required.
6. Inject directly into the tissue to be anaesthetised such as the edge of a wound or the skin overlying the site of a lesion to be excised. Alternatively, a field block can be achieved by injecting around the perimeter of the region to be anaesthetised (Figure 5.3).

For certain procedures, blocking the supplying sensory nerves to the area is an effective technique which requires thorough anatomical knowledge regarding the course of these nerves. Examples include:

A digital block (Figure 5.4): Inject 2–3 mL of solution into both sides of the affected finger starting along the dorsal skin just distal to the metacarpal-phalangeal (MCP) and aim towards the MCP joint in a volar direction. This will block the two digital nerves which travel on the medial and lateral sides of the digits.

Supraorbital nerve block (Figure 5.5): This is used for anaesthetising the medial upper eyelid, medial nose and upper forehead. After injecting the superficial tissue, advance the needle toward the exit of the nerve from the skull located between the medial third and lateral two-thirds of the palpated supraorbital rim and inject the remaining anaesthetic.

Anatomical pitfalls

Adrenaline should be avoided in digital blocks, distal organs (such as the penis, fingers, toes, and earlobes), areas of poor vascular supply, and contaminated wounds due to the risk of infection.

Top tips

- Using sodium bicarbonate as a buffer (included in the preparation) has been shown to decrease the painful sting caused by lidocaine by increasing the pH of the mixture.
- If there is bleeding and in an area where it is safe to use, adrenaline is often added to minimise the bleeding.
- The longer lasting effect of bupivacaine often makes this the preferable anaesthetic agent in cases where there is commonly postprocedural pain as it provides a greater lasting analgesia effect.

6 Obtaining consent

Francesca Crawley

Figure 6.1 The GMC provides advice on consent, available on their website: https://www.gmc-uk.org/ethical-guidance/ethical-guidance-for-doctors/consent. The Royal College of Surgeons of England also offers guidance on consenting patients, available from https://www.rcseng.ac.uk/library-and-publications/rcs-publications/docs/consent-good-practice-guide/ Copyright The Royal College of Surgeons of England. Reproduced with permission.

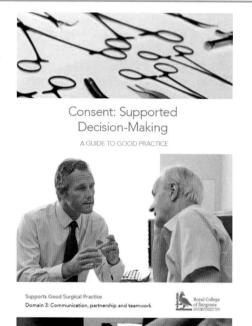

Figure 6.2 Consent forms. Choose the correct form for the procedure and patient.

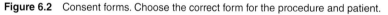

Figure 6.3 Decision making with regard to obtaining consent and which form to use.

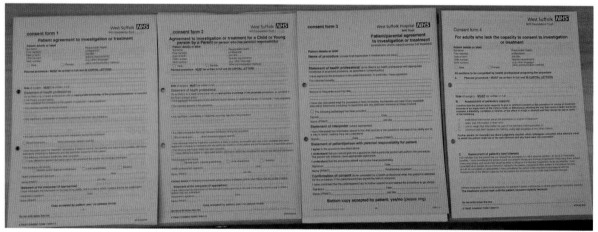

	Major procedure with potential serious complications/side effects or research procedure	**Minor procedure**
Patient has capacity	Written consent Consent form 1 for procedures under general anaesthetic/sedation Consent form 3 for procedures under local anaesthetic	Verbal consent
Patient does not have capacity	Adult: involve family/friends, advance directive; consent form 4 Child: use appropriate language, include carer with parental responsibility; consent form 2	Adult: use appropriate language, proceed in patient's best interest Child: use appropriate language, verbal consent from carer with child

Applied Anatomy for Clinical Procedures at a Glance, First Edition. Jane Sturgess, Francesca Crawley, Ramez Kirollos, and Kirsty Cattle.
© 2021 John Wiley & Sons Ltd. Published 2021 by John Wiley & Sons Ltd.

Why do we obtain consent?

Every decision that involves delivering healthcare to a patient requires consent. This includes treating minor problems, major surgery, and all of the procedures in this book. Obtaining consent is about sharing information and risk with patients and providing them with the information that allows them to understand what will happen to them. Whatever we as practitioners think is the right thing, we must respect the opinion of the patient. (Figure 6.1)

Principles of obtaining consent if the patient has capacity

- Ensure that you understand the procedure that you are asking the patient to consent to. The General Medical Council has clear rules around this: if you cannot do the procedure yourself (such as cardiothoracic surgery) you cannot obtain consent. Do NOT compromise on this.
- Start by discussing with the patient their current health and why any intervention is required.
- Use your specialist knowledge and experience to explain why the procedure you wish to do is in the patient's best interests.
- Explain exactly what the procedure involves and the risks/side effects that could occur. Do not put pressure on the patient to agree to the procedure, even if it seems very obvious to you.
- Allow the patient time to weigh up the advantages and disadvantages of having the procedure. They can then choose whether they will allow it to occur. If there are alternatives, these should also be considered. The patient's decision is final and you cannot override it, whatever you think of it.
- If the patient asks for a procedure or treatment that you do not think is indicated, explain your reasoning behind refusing it. You do not have to provide it, but you must explain why you have come to this decision. Consider offering a second opinion/person for the patient to talk to.

Principles of obtaining consent if the patient does not have capacity

Capacity is the ability to be given information and to retain it for long enough to be able to make a decision based on that information. If patients do not have capacity it may be the case that they have previously expressed an opinion about what they would want to happen in this situation (e.g. major surgery and a likely intensive therapy unit admission) and that should be respected. Otherwise, the opinion of their family, particularly their next of kin, should be respected and a decision reached with them.

Obtaining consent

- You need to explain the procedure honestly, sharing enough information so that the patient understands why you want to do it and the benefit and risk to them.
- If the procedure is part of a research project, this must be explicitly explained and documented.
- The patient may wish to discuss the procedure with a relative or friend, but ultimately the decision to undergo it is theirs and only their consent is valid.
- Explore the patient's concerns and answer these to the best of your ability. If you cannot provide an answer, ask a senior for help.
- Do not withhold information, even if you think it might upset the patient.
- If they do not want to hear about a procedure, explain that you need to inform them before you can do it. Do not perform a procedure without consent. Seek senior help.
- Sometimes your time is limited and you may struggle to provide all the information that the patient wants. Written information provided by your trust may help. Consider involving another member of the healthcare team who understands the procedure.

Responsibility for obtaining consent

This should lie with the doctor doing the procedure. If they cannot obtain consent from the patient, for whatever reason (e.g. time), they can delegate, providing this is to someone who is capable of doing the procedure themselves.

Discussing side effects/risk

You should provide clear and accurate information about the risk, side effects, and complications of a procedure, including the risk of not having it. Use clear language and check understanding.

Verbal or written consent? (Figures 6.2 and 6.3)

- For minor procedures (such as venesection or arterial blood gases) verbal consent is generally sufficient, particularly as the patient is able to demonstrate their consent by, for example, offering their arm.
- For more major procedures always check the trust policy and, if in doubt, obtain written consent. Written consent is always required if the procedure is for research.

Consent in children

- You should do your best to explain any procedure to a child. If they are over 16 they generally have capacity and some children younger than this may also. It is always sensible to include a parent or next of kin, and this is mandatory if the child does not have capacity.

7 Manometer for central venous pressure and lumbar puncture

Jane Sturgess

Figure 7.1 A simple manometer line.

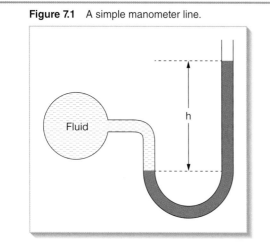

Figure 7.2 Standard CSF manometer line; note the hollow tube, connected to the patient via the spinal needle and three-way tap (a), and the cm markings along the manometer tube (b). The manometer must be kept vertical and the reading taken from the top of the meniscus.

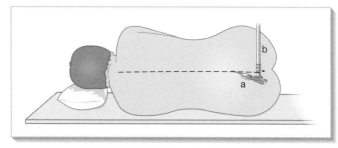

Figure 7.3 Standard CVP manometer line showing the continuous column of fluid (a) attached to the patient's circulation, the transducer (b) that changes the pressure generated by the patient's blood into an electronic signal to produce a waveform on the monitor.

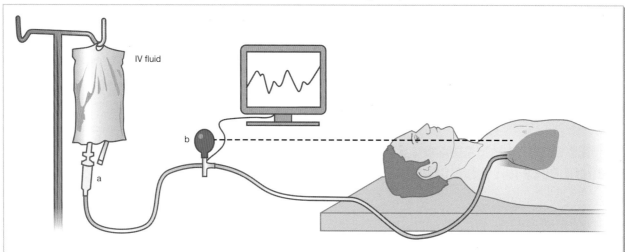

Figure 7.4 CSF manometer and three-way tap setup.

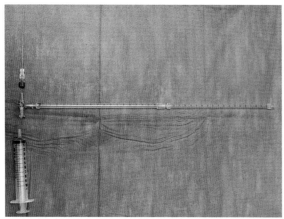

Figure 7.5 Equipment required for CVP.

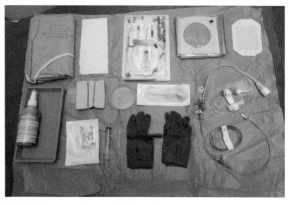

Applied Anatomy for Clinical Procedures at a Glance, First Edition. Jane Sturgess, Francesca Crawley, Ramez Kirollos, and Kirsty Cattle.
© 2021 John Wiley & Sons Ltd. Published 2021 by John Wiley & Sons Ltd.

What is a manometer line?

A manometer measures pressure. In clinical circumstances this is the pressure difference between a clinical variable (CVP, CSF pressure) and the atmosphere (also known as gauge pressure).

In its simplest form it is measured by assessing how high a column of fluid (blood or CSF) can be driven (by the patients' own internal physiological pressure) up a hollow tube that is connected to the patients' blood or cerebrospinal fluid (CSF), which is open to air at the opposite end (Figure 7.1). The height of this column of fluid is measured in cmH_2O. This is the manometer line most commonly used for CSF opening and closing pressures (Figure 7.2). Central venous pressure (CVP) is more commonly measured using a transducer that transmits the pressure generated on a column of fluid (blood from a central vein to a continuous column of saline) into an electronic signal that gives a waveform on a monitor (Figure 7.3).

What is normal pressure?

- CVP is given a normal pressure range of 0–15 cmH_2O.
- CSF pressure is normally 10–20 cmH_2O.

Set-up of the CSF manometer line

Equipment (Figure 7.4)

- Three-way tap
- Spinal needle
- CSF manometer line (plus a spare if you think CSF pressure will be very high)

Technique

1. Attach the three-way tap to the manometer line and turn the tap to face away from the manometer line.
2. Perform lumbar puncture.
3. Attach the three-way tap to the lumen of the spinal needle. Turn the three-way tap so that it is open to the patient and manometer and closed to air.
4. Watch the fluid column rise until it stops. This is the opening pressure. There are natural oscillations with respiration.
5. Note how much CSF you remove (if any) to bring the CSF pressure to within normal limits. Note the closing pressure.

Set-up of the CVP manometer line

Equipment (Figure 7.5)

- CVP line
- 500 mL N. saline
- Pressure bag
- Pressure transducer 'giving' set
- Monitoring cable
- Monitor

Technique

1. Attach the pressure transducer 'giving' set to the bag of saline and flush the system through ensuring there are no air bubbles.
2. Pressurise the bag of saline to 300 mmHg (so that it is guaranteed to be higher than systolic pressure and permit a continuous column of saline with no back flow of blood).
3. Connect the transducer to the monitor with the monitoring line.
4. Check that when the line is flushed the monitor registers >200 mmHg, and that when it is open to air it registers 0 mmHg.
5. Perform CVP line.
6. Attach the manometer line to the distal port of the CVP line.
7. Zero the line at the monitor by turning the three-way tap so that it is closed to the patient but open to air. A zero means atmospheric pressure is 0 mmHg.
8. Flush the system.
9. Continuously measure the CVP, ensuring consistent placement of the transducer. It is standard practice to place the transducer at the height of the right atrium (manubriosternal angle) to measure right atrial central venous pressure.

Common anatomical pitfalls

CSF

1. Sitting position – as pressure is measured in cmH_2O a sitting pressure will be greater than a lying pressure. This must be noted.
2. Clot in the line – aspirate and flush. A clot will not permit free flow of the column of fluid. CSF is less dense than blood and will rise further.
3. Avoid using extra manometer line as this may cause dependent loops and cause inaccurate readings. Stick to three-way taps and manometer line.

CVP

1. Poor zeroing technique. With an electronic transducer the pressure measurement gained will be completely dependent upon the level of the transducer. It should be placed at the level of the patient's right atrium.
2. Using the number – the number may vary according to patient pathology. The most important factor is the trend in the numbers rather than the numbers themselves.
3. Bubbles in the giving set can cause abnormal pressure readings – ensure a bubble-free system.
4. A loss of pressure in the system will cause inaccurate readings.

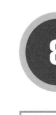

8

Bladder irrigation sets

Jane Sturgess

Figure 8.1 Setting up the irrigation set. The set is primed from a single irrigation bag, whilst the second port remains clamped shut. Note the clamped lumen (a) and the shut flow switch (b). The height of the drip stand is no more than a meter above bed height.

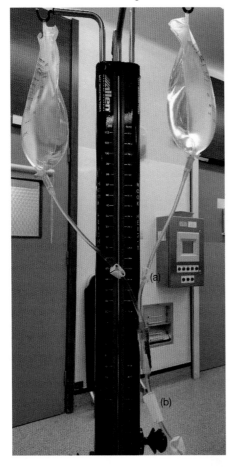

Figure 8.3 The entire irrigation set-up. (a) Open the flow switches on the primed section of the irrigation set – keep them shut/clamped on the redundant arm, (b) check fluid is dripping in the fluid chamber of the giving set, (c) monitor hourly urine output and the amount of irrigation fluid used. Urine output = total output – irrigation fluid used.

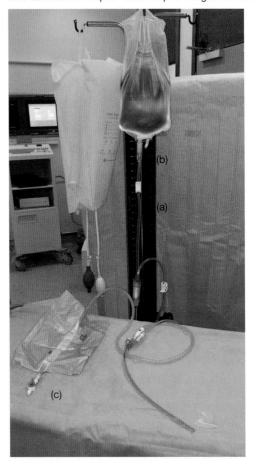

Figure 8.2 Attaching the irrigation and catheter bag to the catheter. (a) Attach the catheter bag to the middle port of the three-way catheter, (b) check urine flows, (c) attach the irrigation to the second wide lumen, (d) the third port is to inflate the balloon of the urinary catheter. A spigot (e) may be used if haematuria clears and irrigation is no longer required – remove the irrigation fluid and place the spigot in the second wide lumen.

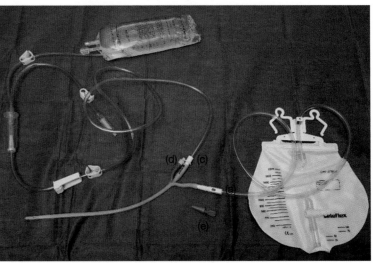

Applied Anatomy for Clinical Procedures at a Glance, First Edition. Jane Sturgess, Francesca Crawley, Ramez Kirollos, and Kirsty Cattle.
© 2021 John Wiley & Sons Ltd. Published 2021 by John Wiley & Sons Ltd.

Equipment

- Equipment for catheterisation (see Chapter 10)
- 1–2 litres irrigation fluid (often normal saline)
- 3x 10 mL syringes filled with water
- Irrigation tubing (with an integral Y connector)
- Three-way Foley catheter and stand
- 4-litre Foley catheter bag (to hold urine and irrigation fluid)

Set-up

1. Prime your irrigation set in the same way that you would set up an IV line, and then turn the flow switch off and clamp the lumen shut (Figure 8.1). Hang it on a drip stand at not greater than 1 meter above the height of the patient's bed. NB. Prime the system only from 1 of the irrigation bags, whilst the second side remains clamped shut.
2. Open your catheter bag making sure you keep the connector that attaches to the urinary catheter sterile.
3. Attach the catheter bag to the middle port of the three-way Foley catheter.
4. Remove the protective cover from the end of the irrigation set (all the way to the white tip) and attach the irrigation tubing to the second lumen of the three-way Foley catheter (Figure 8.2).
5. Insert the urinary catheter (see Chapter 10 for males or 11 for females).
6. Use all 30 mL of saline to inflate the balloon of the urinary catheter.
7. Check urine flows into the bag; a clot may obstruct flow.
8. Once you have confirmed flow of urine, open the irrigation flow switch and unclamp the lumen attached to irrigation fluid. If the second lumen is not attached to irrigation fluid it must remain clamped.
9. Check that you can see irrigation fluid dripping in the drip chamber – this indicates flow towards the patient's bladder. Then check urine is flowing into the catheter bag (Figure 8.3).
10. Monitor the hourly urine output – it is important to maintain a strict input/output fluid balance.
11. Bladder irrigation usually continues until the urine is rosé coloured or clear.

Common anatomical pitfalls

- No urine flow – either the catheter is not in the bladder (or has created a false urethral passage) or a clot is obstructing the flow. The clot can be in the urinary catheter or over the Foley catheter opening.

Top tips

- Do not use water as an irrigation fluid. This can be absorbed into the circulation and cause a dilutional hyponatraemia.
- Suspect a blocked catheter if the patient complains of suprapubic or lower abdominal pain and becomes sweaty, tachycardic, and hypotensive. Stop the irrigation fluid and consider manual bladder irrigation.
- Recatheterisation can be difficult – ask for help.
- Manual irrigation – if the catheter stops draining, it may be blocked with clots. Manual irrigation is required to break up the clots and clear the catheter. Stop the irrigation and spigot the second wide lumen. Use a catheter syringe to infiltrate 50 mL of saline in through the drainage lumen. To empty the bladder and remove the clots, either use gentle suction on the syringe to drain the bladder or allow it to drain freely by disconnecting the bladder syringe and allowing the catheter to drain into a kidney bowl or reattach the drainage bag and hang it below the level of the patient. Continue until all clots have been removed (no further clots in drained urine) then reconnect the irrigation at a faster rate than previously to reduce risk of further clots forming.

9 Underwater seal for chest drains

Jane Sturgess

Figure 9.1 Equipment.

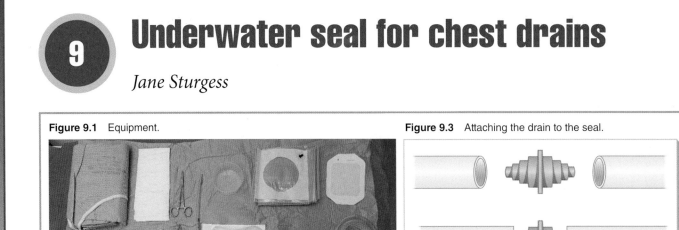

Figure 9.3 Attaching the drain to the seal.

Figure 9.2 (a) single, (b) double, (c) triple chamber underwater seals. The combined triple chamber drain is most frequently used.

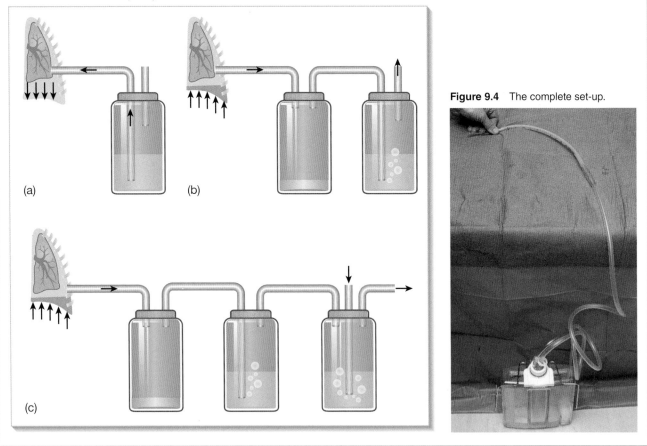

(a)

(b)

(c)

Figure 9.4 The complete set-up.

Applied Anatomy for Clinical Procedures at a Glance, First Edition. Jane Sturgess, Francesca Crawley, Ramez Kirollos, and Kirsty Cattle.
© 2021 John Wiley & Sons Ltd. Published 2021 by John Wiley & Sons Ltd.

Equipment (Figure 9.1)

Also see Chapter 21, Intercostal drains.

- Sterile drainage system. There are a number of different types available: single, double, or triple chamber (Figure 9.2).
- Sterile water to fill to zero line in the water seal chamber (check manufacturers volume required) and to the 20 cm level in the suction control chamber (if used)
- Waterproof adhesive tape, for example, Leukoplast Sleek (NB this contains latex)
- Chest drain container (to permit it to be fixed to the bedside)
- Oxygen supply (include portable if transferring the patient between clinical areas)
- Low pressure suction max 10 KPa (include portable if transferring the patient between clinical areas)

Connection (Figures 9.3 and 9.4)

The chest drain and the drainage system often connect via a female:female connector. A firm push and twist are often sufficient; however, some clinicians recommend the use of tape at this connection point to prevent accidental disconnection and resultant air leak. The tape can be circumferential or longitudinal. The proposed benefit of longitudinal tape is that it permits the nursing staff to make a visual inspection of the integrity of the connection during their post-procedure observations.

How does it work? (see Figure 9.2)

1. The water level acts as a one-way valve – only permitting air/fluid to flow from the intrapleural cavity during expiration and barring backflow despite the subatmospheric pressures generated during the inspiratory cycle.
2. Minimum requirements are (i) an underwater seal, (ii) a collection chamber, (iii) low resistance circuit.
3. The circuit may be passive (relying purely on gravity and the pressures generated during the respiratory cycle) or active (by the application of suction to remove fluid/air from the intrapleural space and reinflate the lung).

Anatomical pitfalls

1. Reaccumulation or tensioning of a pneumothorax can occur if the chest drain becomes deliberately (clamped) or inadvertently occluded, and air continues to leak from the parietal pleura into the pleural cavity. If your patient suddenly becomes breathless check for clamps, kinking of the drainage tubing (including being caught in the side-rails of the bed), or clot.
2. Persistent pneumothorax and/or symptoms. Arrange a chest X-ray to check the position of the chest drain. Apical pneumothoraces require a drain directed towards the apex of the lung.
3. Loculated air or fluid collections can be difficult to drain and may require multiple chest drains often sited under ultrasound guidance. Consider this if there is no resolution of the effusion/empyema even if the chest X-ray suggests a correctly placed drain.
4. Incorrect fluid level in the drainage system – too low. A tachypnoeic, distressed patient may generate a negative intrapleural pressure up to -80 cmH$_2$0. If the fluid level is only 1 cm above the end of the drainage tube the patient becomes at risk of air aspiration from the drainage system on inspiration.
5. Incorrect fluid level in the drainage system – too high (single chamber). Gravity and forced expiration and coughing (generating a positive intrapleural pressure) are important in allowing free drainage of fluid/empyema/blood/air from the intrapleural space. A high fluid level in the drainage system requires the generation of higher pressures and results in less drainage.
6. Dependent loops of tubing between the drainage system and the patient can fill with fluid and cause similar problems to 5.
7. Zero level of the collection system at or above the insertion point of the chest drain. As the patient generates a negative intrapleural pressure gradient at the start of inspiration, fluid will be drawn up the drain towards the pleural cavity. This is especially important in patients with obstructed ventilation who can generate up to -80 cmH$_2$0 subatmospheric pressure on inspiration. The drain needs to be placed 100 cm below the level of the chest drain insertion point. It can cause two problems: (i) inadequate drainage of intrapleural pathology, and (ii) potential for fluid, clot, infected material to enter the intrapleural cavity from the drainage system (siphoning).
8. Beware of the drainage system being placed higher than the patient, especially during transfer, causing fluid to re-enter the pleural cavity.
9. Suction applied at greater than 10 KPa can traumatise the tissues by trapping lung tissue into the eyelets of the chest drain. The drain will also fail to work as the system is occluded.

Top tips

- Bubbling of the fluid in the chest drainage system on expiration indicates that the chest tube is in the pleural space, that the system is patent throughout, and that a draining pneumothorax is still present. Persistent bubbling throughout the respiratory cycle indicates a bronchopleural fistula.
- A swinging fluid level during normal respiration and after a deep breath indicates that the chest tube is in the pleural space and that the system is patent throughout.
- When closing the drain consider placing the clamp on the patient side of the female:female connection. If there is an inadvertent disconnection the drain will remain closed. The drain can be clamped for two main reasons: (i) to assess how well the patient will tolerate removal of the drain (even if there is a small residual pneumothorax), and (ii) to facilitate retention of medication in the intrapleural space after therapeutic injection.
- If the drain stops bubbling or swinging it can mean either (i) the lung has reinflated and the pneumothorax or haemothorax is resolved/treated, (ii) the drain has become displaced and is no longer in the intrapleural space, (iii) loss of suction (if used), or (iv) the system is no longer patent. You should check for a clamped tube or a clot.
- An indelible marker can be used to mark the time, date, and amount of fluid drained on the bottle to act as a visual trigger of large losses in short time periods. Immediate drainage of more than 500 mL pleural effusion can cause negative pressure pulmonary oedema. More than 500 mL blood loss per hour requires urgent medical review.
- The drain should be changed if more than 500 mL fluid has collected. Volumes greater than this can affect the suction that has been applied.

10 Male catheterisation

Francesca Crawley

Figure 10.1 Equipment required.

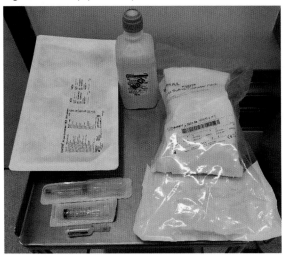

Figure 10.2 Patient positioning and draping.

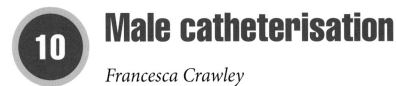

Figure 10.3 Insertion of the catheter. Holding the penis in your non-dominant hand and using the catheter packaging allows an aseptic, non-touch insertion technique which minimises introduction of infection.

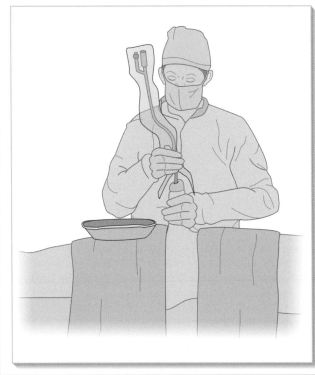

Figure 10.4 Male urethral anatomy.

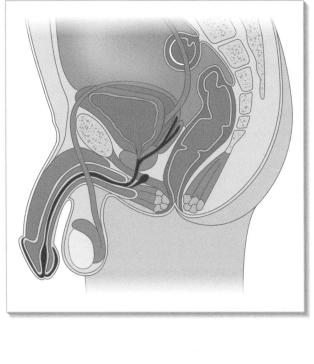

Applied Anatomy for Clinical Procedures at a Glance, First Edition. Jane Sturgess, Francesca Crawley, Ramez Kirollos, and Kirsty Cattle.
© 2021 John Wiley & Sons Ltd. Published 2021 by John Wiley & Sons Ltd.

Equipment (Figure 10.1)

- A catheterisation pack
- A 12–14 Fr male Foley catheter
- A catheter bag
- Sterile gloves
- Antiseptic cleaning fluid
- Lignocaine gel
- A 10 mL syringe filled with sterile water (check the catheter packaging for volume of water the balloon will hold, three-way catheter balloons hold 30 mL of water)

Procedure

1. You need a chaperone.
2. Introduce yourself to the patient and explain what you are going to do.
3. Check for allergies (lignocaine gel, latex).
4. Obtain verbal consent.
5. Position the patient as flat as possible on his back on the bed. His legs should be slightly apart.
6. Using aseptic technique (see Chapter 2) open the catheterisation pack and the catheter. Put the catheter on the sterile surface.
7. Pour antiseptic fluid into the container.
8. Wash your hands and put on the sterile gloves.
9. Drape the patient so that his upper thighs are covered with a sterile drape, his penis is on top of the drape and another drape covers his lower abdomen (Figure 10.2). There may be a fenestrated drape in the pack, in which case place this over the penis without touching the penis.
10. Put a collecting dish (e.g. kidney-shaped dish) between his legs.
11. Hold the penis with a sterile swab and clean the meatus (including around the retracted foreskin).
12. Using a piece of gauze, hold the penis about 4 cm from the meatus.
13. Insert the lignocaine gel into the meatus. This takes about 5 minutes to work. Explain this to the patient.
14. Partially open the plastic bag containing the catheter to reveal the catheter tip.
15. Hold the penis vertically with your non-dominant hand and the plastic bag containing the catheter with the other.
16. Avoiding touching the catheter, advance it into the meatus (Figure 10.3).
17. Whilst still holding the penis via the sterile gauze, continue to advance the catheter until the bifurcation reaches the penis.
18. The catheter passes through the external urethral meatus to the spongy (penile) urethra within the corpus spongiosum, then the membranous urethra which is the segment passing through the perineal membrane or urogenital diaphragm – 'sphincter urethrae', then the prostatic urethra and through the internal urethral orifice in the trigone of the bladder. Within the prostatic urethra a fold – 'urethral crest', harbours the opening of the prostatic utricle and on either side the orifices of the ejaculatory ducts. The spongy urethra has two areas of relative dilatations one at the glans and the other at the bulb (Figure 10.4).
19. Urine should now flow into the collecting dish.
20. Attach the syringe containing sterile water to the catheter and inflate the balloon. This should be painless. If the patient experiences pain deflate the balloon and advance the catheter forwards. Then try inflating the balloon again.
21. Attach the catheter bag.
22. Gently pull back the catheter until resistance is felt. The catheter is now resting on the bladder wall/urethral exit point.
23. Remove the plastic catheter cover by tearing it lengthways along the perforation.
24. Replace the foreskin.
25. Ensure that the patient is clean and dry.
26. Record how much urine initially drains (in the notes and on the observations chart).
27. Dispose of equipment and ensure the patient is comfortable and not exposed.
28. Record the procedure in the patient notes, including the indication and that consent was obtained.

Contraindications

- Lack of consent
- Blood at meatus tip prior to attempting catheterisation. This may indicate trauma. Seek senior advice.
- Known urethral stricture

Common problems

- The catheter does not advance smoothly. If this occurs, gently increase the traction on the penis and rotate the catheter a little. If you cannot advance the catheter, ask for senior help and if none is immediately available, abandon the procedure.
- The foreskin is not replaced adequately. This can lead to a medical emergency as the retracted foreskin becomes swollen and oedematous.

Female catheterisation

11

Francesca Crawley

Figure 11.1 Equipment required.

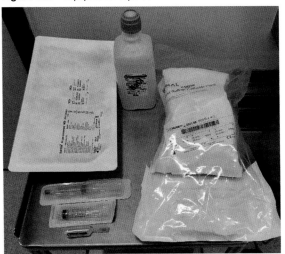

Figure 11.2 Patient positioning.

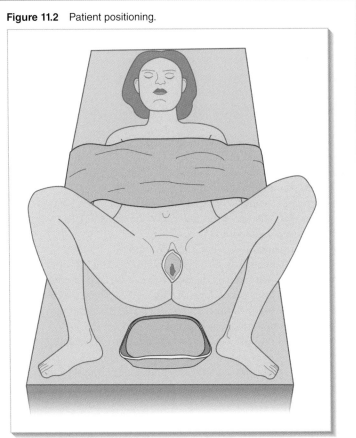

Figure 11.3 Female perineal anatomy.

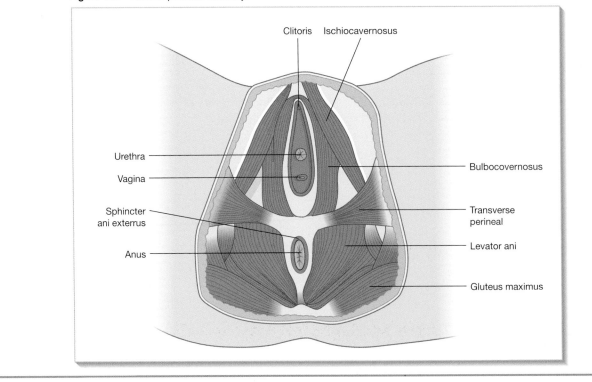

Clitoris   Ischiocavernosus

Urethra

Vagina

Sphincter
ani exterrus

Anus

Bulbocovernosus

Transverse
perineal

Levator ani

Gluteus maximus

Applied Anatomy for Clinical Procedures at a Glance, First edition. Jane Sturgess, Francesca Crawley, Ramez Kirollos, and Kirsty Cattle.
© 2021 John Wiley & Sons Ltd. Published 2021 by John Wiley & Sons Ltd.

Figure 11.4 Female pelvic anatomy.

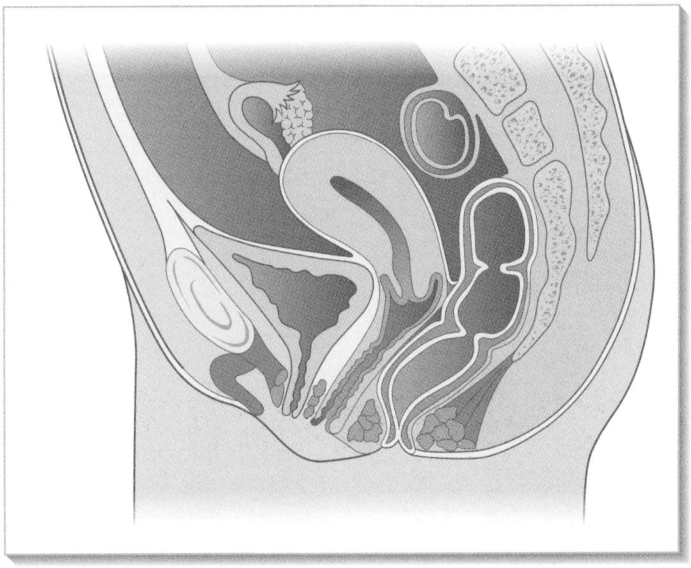

Indications

Female catheterisation is done for

- Urinary retention
- Acute kidney injury (AKI) where urine volume is important

Equipment (Figure 11.1)

- A catheterisation pack
- A 12–14 Fr Foley catheter (male or female)
- A catheter bag
- Sterile gloves
- Antiseptic cleaning fluid
- Lignocaine gel
- A 10 mL syringe filled with sterile water (check the catheter packaging for volume of water the balloon will hold, three-way catheter balloons hold 30 mL of water)

Pre-procedure

1. Check the patient's identity, explain the procedure, and gain her consent.
2. Find a chaperone.

Procedure

1. Position her as flat as possible (Figure 11.2).
2. Ask her to put her ankles together and allow her knees to flop outwards.
3. Using an aseptic technique open the catheter pack and pour aseptic fluid into the receiver.
4. Open the rest of the equipment onto the sterile field.
5. Wash and dry your hands and put on the sterile gloves.
6. Drape the patient and put a collecting vessel between her legs.
7. With your non-dominant hand, part the labia.
8. With your dominant hand clean the urinary meatus with saline-soaked balls, using a single downwards motion with each ball.
9. Ensure you can identify the meatus and keep the labia parted (Figure 11.3).
10. Insert the whole tube of lignocaine gel. Warn the patient that this may be uncomfortable and will take 5 minutes to work.
11. Pick up the catheter with your right hand and start to insert into the meatus until the end arm reaches the meatus. Urine should start to flow.
12. Check the packaging for the exact volume of water needed to inflate the balloon and insert this.
13. Attach the catheter bag.
14. Gently pull on the catheter until resistance is felt. The balloon should now be resting at the urethral opening.
15. Dispose of gloves and equipment in the clinical waste bin. Wash your hands.
16. Record the procedure, including indication and volume of urine in the patient's notes.

Top tips

- Before you introduce the catheter, ask the patient to take a few deep breaths. This will help her to relax and make the procedure easier for you.
- Be sure of the anatomy before introducing the catheter (see Figures 11.3 and 11.4).
- In an elderly woman, if the urethral meatus cannot be identified, it may be on the anterior vaginal wall. It has a firm feeling. With the patient's consent, introduce a finger into the vagina to feel the meatus, advance the catheter along your finger, and feed it into the meatus.

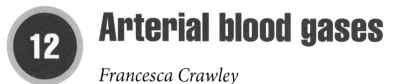

12 Arterial blood gases

Francesca Crawley

Figure 12.1 Equipment required.

Figure 12.2 Anatomy of the radial artery at the wrist.

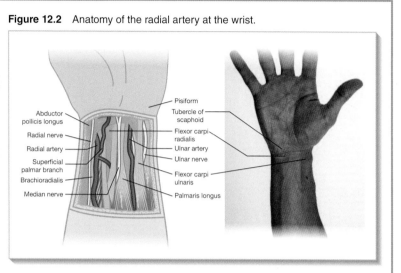

Abductor pollicis longus
Radial nerve
Radial artery
Superficial palmar branch
Brachioradialis
Median nerve

Pisiform
Tubercle of scaphoid
Flexor carpi radialis
Ulnar artery
Ulnar nerve
Flexor carpi ulnaris
Palmaris longus

Figure 12.3 Allen's test. (a) Anatomy of the superficial and deep palmar arches. (b) Ask the patient to clench their fist. (c) Palpate and occlude both radial and ulnar arteries. (d) Ask the patient to relax the hand. The palm should be blanched (white). (e) Then release the pressure on the ulnar artery. The hand should become pink again.

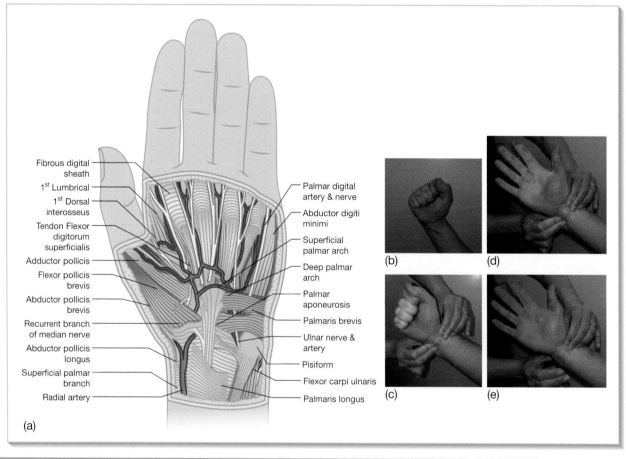

Fibrous digital sheath
1st Lumbrical
1st Dorsal interosseus
Tendon Flexor digitorum superficialis
Adductor pollicis
Flexor pollicis brevis
Abductor pollicis brevis
Recurrent branch of median nerve
Abductor pollicis longus
Superficial palmar branch
Radial artery

Palmar digital artery & nerve
Abductor digiti minimi
Superficial palmar arch
Deep palmar arch
Palmar aponeurosis
Palmaris brevis
Ulnar nerve & artery
Pisiform
Flexor carpi ulnaris
Palmaris longus

(a)
(b)
(c)
(d)
(e)

Applied Anatomy for Clinical Procedures at a Glance, First Edition. Jane Sturgess, Francesca Crawley, Ramez Kirollos, and Kirsty Cattle.

Figure 12.4 Brachial artery anatomy.

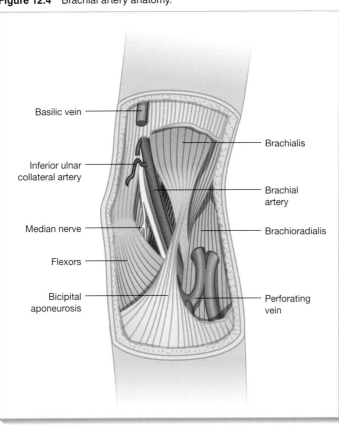

Figure 12.5 Femoral artery anatomy.

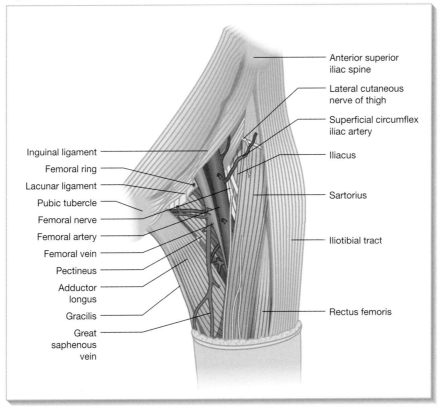

Equipment and procedures for performing arterial blood gas sampling:

Equipment (Figure 12.1)

- Pre-heparinised syringe
- Needles, 20, 23, and 25 gauge
- A bung and cap for the needle and syringe (1–3 are usually provided in an arterial blood gas pack)
- Sharps bin
- Wipe to clean skin, gloves, gauze to cover site, and tape
- Assistant to apply pressure on site post sampling (if patient unable to do this for themselves)

Procedure

Identify patient and assemble equipment

1. Check it is the correct patient by asking them to state their name. Check whether they are on any blood thinning medication (generally warfarin or aspirin).
2. Establish which artery you will draw blood from. The options are radial, brachial, and femoral. Try the radial first and locate it by palpation. Identify relevant local surface anatomy. It overlies the distal radius bone. At the wrist the radial artery is lateral to the tendon of the flexor carpi radialis (Figure 12.2).
3. Wash hands and apply gloves.
4. Perform Allen's test to ensure adequate collateral flow (see right column).
5. Disinfect the patient's skin over the radial artery.
6. Extend the wrist: a pillow may be useful.
7. Assemble needle and syringe. These are generally pre-assembled.
8. Pull the plunger back to the point recommended by the local laboratory.
9. Explain to the patient that you are about to start.

Perform procedure

1. Re-palpate the artery and keep your fingers on it. Press vertically down to obtain the maximum point of pulsation. Press lightly, or you will occlude the artery.
2. Holding the syringe like a dart, steady your hand on the patient's wrist and approach at 45 degrees to the skin with the bevel facing up. Aim towards the maximum point of pulsation. Advance the needle until you see a flashback of blood.
3. Allow the syringe to fill. Do not pull the plunger.
4. Once the arterial blood has reached the predetermined level in the syringe (usually about a centimetre) withdraw the needle, cover it with the bung, and dispose of it. Cap the syringe.

Post-procedure

1. Cover the site with gauze and ask the patient or your assistant to press for about three minutes. This will need to be about five minutes if the patient is anticoagulated.
2. Transport immediately to the lab, on ice if possible.
3. Thank the patient and check that bleeding has ceased. If not, someone needs to continue to press on the puncture point.

Allen's test (Figure 12.3)

This test is to ensure collateral flow before attempting a radial artery puncture. This is provided through the superficial palmar arch (covered only by skin and palmar aponeurosis). It is formed mainly by the ulnar artery with a smaller contribution from the radial artery at the level of the web of the thumb. The radial artery is the main contributor of the deep palmar arch (just distal to the carpal bones) which lies 1–2 cm proximal and deep to the superficial arch. Palpate and occlude both radial and ulnar arteries and ask the patient to clench their fist and then release it. The palm should be blanched (white). Then release the pressure on the ulnar artery. The hand should become pink again. This implies that there is good collateral circulation and even if you were to damage the radial artery, the hand would be perfused via the ulnar.

Brachial and femoral stabs

These arteries are bigger and in theory may be easier to obtain arterial blood from. However, in practice, they are deeper and harder to palpate. They are surrounded by crucial structures, which can be easily damaged.

The brachial artery is related to the medial aspect of the humerus proximally and anterior to it more distally. It is separated from the superficially lying median cubital vein by the bicipital aponeurosis. At the elbow the median nerve is just medial to the brachial artery. It bifurcates into radial and ulnar arteries about 2–3 cm below the crease of the elbow (Figure 12.4).

The femoral artery lies in the femoral triangle below the inguinal ligament occupying the lateral compartment of the femoral sheath (the femoral vein is in the middle compartment and the medial compartment contains lymph vessels/lymph node of Cloquet and is the 'femoral canal'. The femoral nerve is lateral to the femoral sheath). It is covered by skin subcutaneous tissue and fascia lata. Its surface marking is midpoint between the anterior superior iliac spine and the pubic tubercle (Figure 12.5).

Haematomas are also more common. It is harder to obtain haemostasis. Obtaining arterial blood gases from these arteries is generally second line, if the brachial is impossible or the patient uncooperative and moving (when the femoral, being more fixed in the groin, may be a better option).

Common anatomical pitfalls

- Unable to draw blood from radial artery:
  - Withdraw syringe a little and reinsert in a slightly different direction.
  - Try this twice and then abandon that artery and move to the other radial artery or to a brachial or femoral artery.
  - Consider asking for help. Arterial blood gases are an uncomfortable procedure for the patient.
- Bleeding from puncture site does not stop: Continue to press on the puncture site until it does. Ask someone else to do this if necessary.

Top tips

- Explain to the patient that the procedure is uncomfortable. They are then less likely to flinch during the procedure.
- Establish how to get the sample to the analyser before you start.
- Alert another member of staff before you start that you may need help pressing on the puncture site.

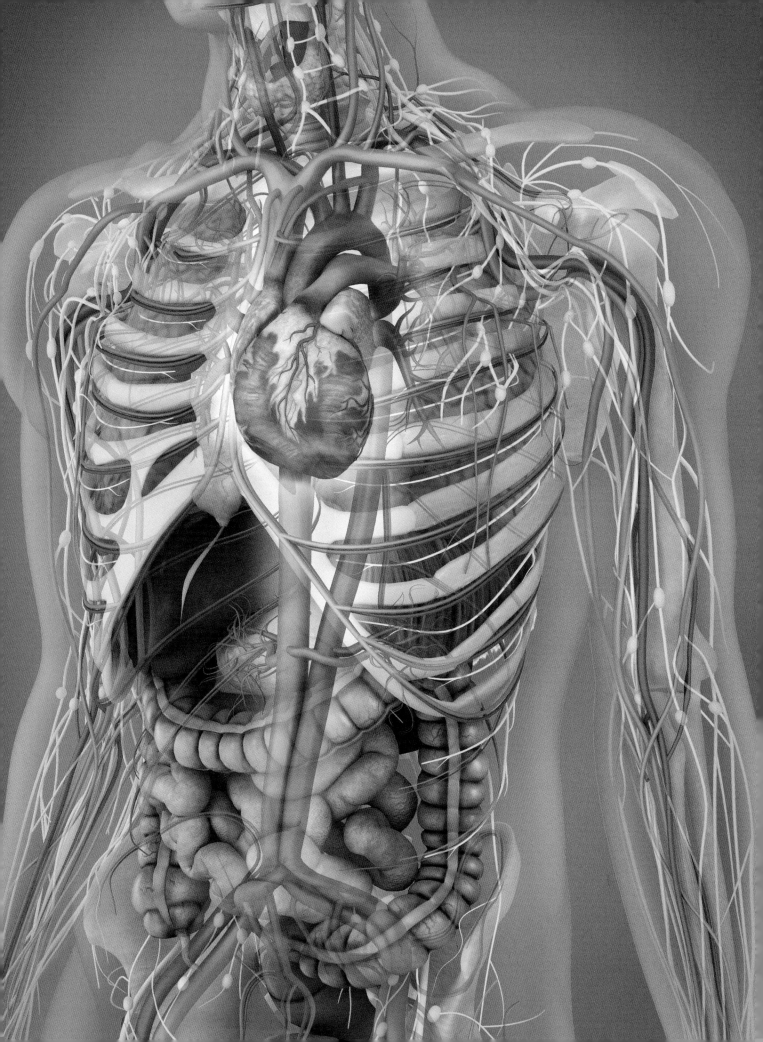

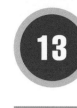

13 Performing an electrocardiogram

Francesca Crawley

Figure 13.1 Equipment required.

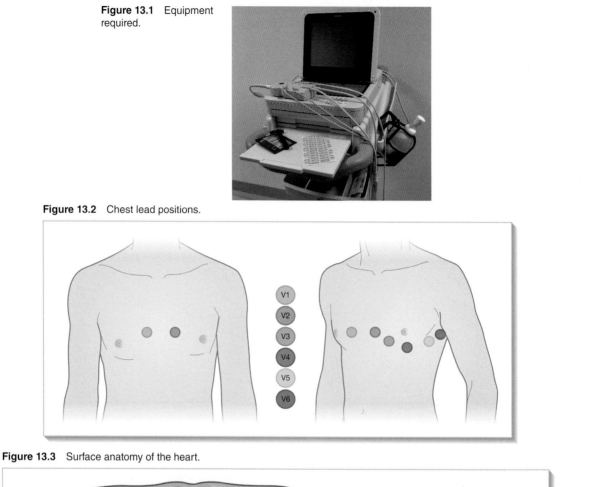

Figure 13.2 Chest lead positions.

V1
V2
V3
V4
V5
V6

Figure 13.3 Surface anatomy of the heart.

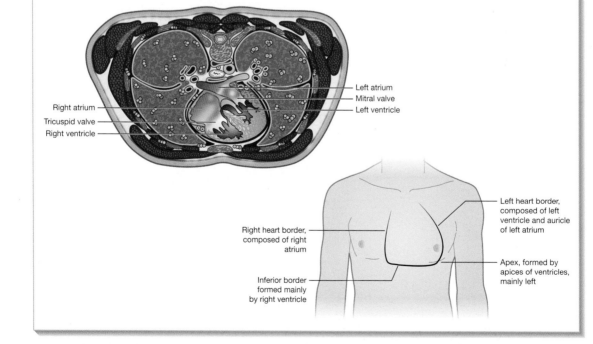

Left atrium
Mitral valve
Left ventricle

Right atrium
Tricuspid valve
Right ventricle

Left heart border, composed of left ventricle and auricle of left atrium

Right heart border, composed of right atrium

Apex, formed by apices of ventricles, mainly left

Inferior border formed mainly by right ventricle

Applied Anatomy for Clinical Procedures at a Glance, First Edition. Jane Sturgess, Francesca Crawley, Ramez Kirollos, and Kirsty Cattle.
© 2021 John Wiley & Sons Ltd. Published 2021 by John Wiley & Sons Ltd.

Equipment (Figure 13.1)
- Electrocardiogram (ECG) machine
- 10 sticky pads
- Hand sanitizer
- Razor

Procedure
1. Expose the patient's chest. A chaperone may be necessary. You may need to shave the chest if it is very hairy.
2. Apply the sticky pads as follows:
   a. One to the inner surface of both wrists
   b. One to each ankle
   c. Six across the chest (Figure 13.2):
      - V1 at right sternal border
      - V2 at left sternal border
      - V3 between V2 and V4
      - V4 in fifth intercostal space, midclavicular line
      - V5 horizontal to V4 in anterior axillary line
      - V6 horizontal to V4 and V5 in midaxillary line

   In relationship to the anterior chest wall, anatomically, the right border of the heart is formed mainly by the right atrium, the inferior border by the right ventricle, and the left border by the left ventricle (+a bit by the left atrium). The anterior interventricular sulcus is a thumb's breadth from the left border of the heart.

   The sinoatrial (SA) node is located in the right atrium at the superior end of the sulcus terminalis and the atrioventricular (AV) node at the inferior interatrial septum and continues as the AV bundle which divides into right and left branches (Figure 13.3; see also Figure 37.3).
3. Attach leads to pads.
   a. Start with limb leads and follow traffic light colours (or Ride Your Green Bike):
      - Red to right wrist
      - Yellow to left wrist
      - Green to left ankle
      - Black to right ankle
   b. The chest leads are attached by number (Figure 13.2).
4. Check that the patient is ready to lie still and relaxed for a short period and press 'start' on the ECG machine. If you are unsure where this is, ask a member of staff to show you. If the patient has symptoms (such as chest pain) during the ECG write this on the trace.
5. Ensure the correct patient identification and date is on the ECG and that it is an adequate trace. If in doubt, ask.
6. Remove the leads and ask the patient if they would like you to remove the sticky pads. Most would rather do this themselves.
7. Thank the patient and allow them to get dressed.

Anatomical (and other) pitfalls
1. Sticky pads not fully adherent. Check and replace or reposition.
2. Muscle artefact. If the patient is shivering consider covering them with a light blanket after applying the leads or warm the room.
3. Incorrect placement of limb leads. Recheck before you press 'start'.

Top tips
1. Ensure the patient is warm and relaxed.
2. Ensure good skin-pad contact.
3. Put the leads on correctly and check before you start recording.
4. If you are not familiar with the equipment, find a nurse to help you.
5. Before you start recording, check the leads one more time (especially the limb ones).
6. If pads do not stick, use clinell wipe on the skin and allow to dry and try again.

Oropharyngeal airway

14

Jane Sturgess

Figure 14.1 Equipment.

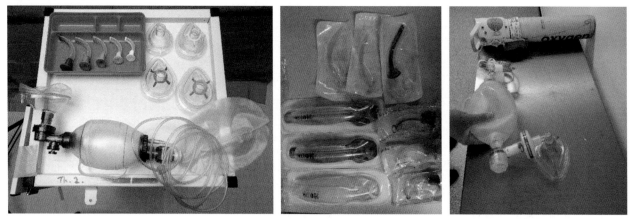

Figure 14.2 Sagittal anatomy of the upper airway.

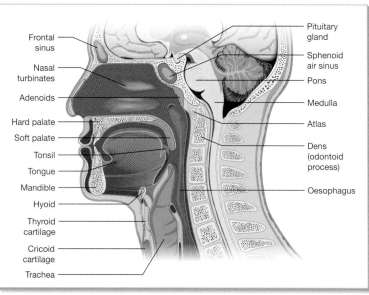

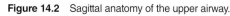

Frontal sinus
Nasal turbinates
Adenoids
Hard palate
Soft palate
Tonsil
Tongue
Mandible
Hyoid
Thyroid cartilage
Cricoid cartilage
Trachea

Pituitary gland
Sphenoid air sinus
Pons
Medulla
Atlas
Dens (odontoid process)
Oesophagus

Figure 14.4 Soft tissue trauma following poorly inserted oropharyngeal airway. Reproduced with permission from Reid et al., published in The Laryngoscope © 2019 The American Laryngological, Rhinological and Otological Society, Inc.

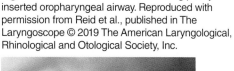

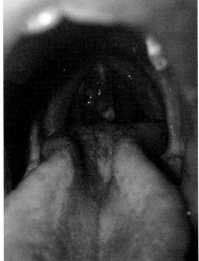

Figure 14.3 Technique oropharyngeal airway: (a) size the airway, (b) open the mouth and insert upside down to the hard palate, (c) rotate 180 degrees and advance the guedel into the airway, (d) 'seating' the airway, with correct position of airway shown.

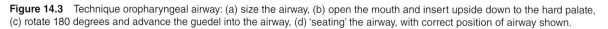
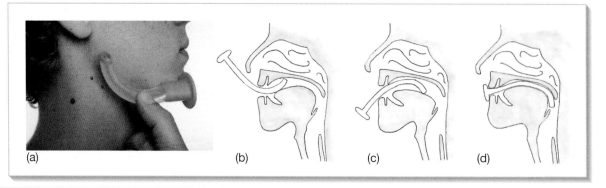

(a) (b) (c) (d)

Applied Anatomy for Clinical Procedures at a Glance, First Edition. Jane Sturgess, Francesca Crawley, Ramez Kirollos, and Kirsty Cattle.
© 2021 John Wiley & Sons Ltd. Published 2021 by John Wiley & Sons Ltd.

Equipment (Figure 14.1)

- Ambu Bag, oxygen tubing
- Oxygen supply – (i) Cylinder – check it is full, they have a dial at the top, the needle should be in the green zone or (ii) Piped – but have a cylinder as backup
- Face masks size 3 (pink ring colour) or 4 (yellow ring colour) ♀, 4 or 5 (green ring colour) ♂
- Oropharyngeal airways size 3, 4, 5
- Nasopharyngeal airways size 6, 7, 8
- Laryngeal mask airway (LMA) size 3, 4, 5 (in case bag mask ventilation is impossible, as a backup)

Technique (Figure 14.2)

Only unconscious patients will tolerate this procedure. If placed in the semi-conscious patient it may induce retching and vomiting and place the airway at risk of contamination.

1. Size the airway. Turn it upside down and place the coloured hub in line with the incisor teeth. The correct size can be determined if the tip of the airway reaches to the tragus (see Figure 14.3a).
2. Stand at the head end of the patient. Pre-oxygenate the patient by supporting the airway and using high flow oxygen. If the patient is not breathing you may need to try and provide 2–3 breaths with a bag mask ventilation system.
3. Open the patient's mouth and remove any debris or vomit under direct vision using a Yankauer sucker.
4. Hold the airway in your right hand and turn it upside down.
5. Introduce the end of the airway into the mouth until the tip is at the border of the hard and soft palate. Rotate the airway through 180 degrees so the curved border now sits against the curve of the tongue.
6. Gently advance the airway into the mouth, displacing the tongue towards the floor of the mouth and away from the soft tissue of the oropharynx.
7. Stop advancing the airway when the coloured hub is in line with the incisors. Sometimes this may require a gentle jaw thrust to enable the airway to 'seat' itself properly (see Figure 14.3).
8. Look, listen, and feel to check that the airway is now patent. Continue to check, and monitor oxygen saturation (SaO_2), respiratory rate, and signs of intolerance of the airway.

Aftercare

1. Place the sedated or unconscious patient in the recovery position so that the airway can be easily cleared if the patient regurgitates or vomits.
2. If the patient starts to cough or choke remove the airway.
3. Ensure the patient is accompanied by a trained person to monitor for continued airway patency until (i) they regain consciousness (if sedated or post seizure), or (ii) help arrives to site a definitive airway.
4. Minimal monitoring includes SaO_2, respiratory rate, and looking, listening, and feeling for airway patency.
5. Remove the airway gently and check for blood on the outer surface. Be prepared for bleeding into the airway.

Common anatomical pitfalls

1. Too big an airway reaches and stimulates the laryngeal inlet, producing coughing, choking, or vomiting.
2. Too big an airway protrudes from the lips. The teeth bite onto the curved portion of the airway, displacing it further. In addition the curve of the airway is designed to mimic the patent oropharynx and displace the posterior border of the tongue anteriorly and into the floor of the mouth – thereby displacing the tongue and reducing the occlusion of the soft tissues.
3. Failing to take care to free the tongue and lips from becoming placed between the airway and the teeth will result in localised tissue trauma.
4. Oral airways can cause lingual nerve damage.
5. Failing to be gentle when rotating the oral airway at the junction of the hard and soft palate can cause local trauma to the soft tissues, including the uvula (Figure 14.4).

Top tips

1. Oral airway sizing – mostly size 3 for small adult female, size 4 for females, size 4 for males, and size 5 for large males.
2. On average it is 12 cm from the teeth to the larynx in women and 14 cm in men.

15 Nasopharyngeal airway

Jane Sturgess

Figure 15.1 Equipment.

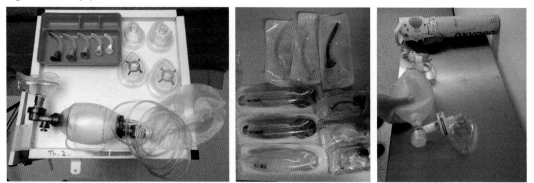

Figure 15.2 Technique nasopharyngeal airway: (a) size the airway, (b) making it safe, (c) insertion, (d) direction to advance the airway.

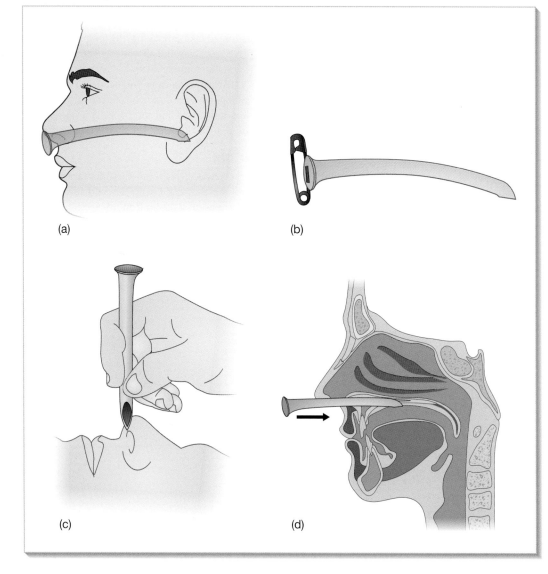

(a)

(b)

(c)

(d)

Applied Anatomy for Clinical Procedures at a Glance, First Edition. Jane Sturgess, Francesca Crawley, Ramez Kirollos, and Kirsty Cattle.
© 2021 John Wiley & Sons Ltd. Published 2021 by John Wiley & Sons Ltd.

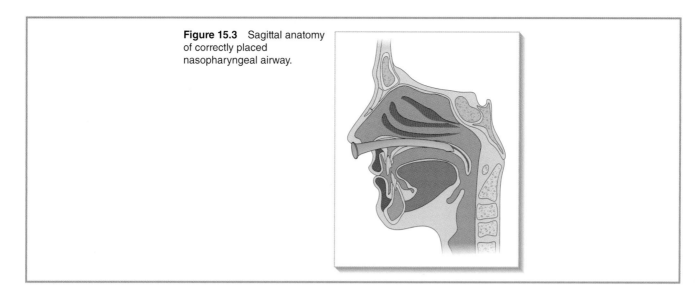

Figure 15.3 Sagittal anatomy of correctly placed nasopharyngeal airway.

Equipment (Figure 15.1)
- Ambu Bag, oxygen tubing
- Oxygen supply – (i) Cylinder – ensure it is full, they have a dial at the top, the needle should be in the green zone or (ii) Piped – but have a cylinder as backup
- Face masks size 3 (pink ring colour) or 4(yellow ring colour) ♀, 4 or 5 (green ring colour) ♂
- Oropharyngeal airways size 3, 4, 5
- Nasopharyngeal airways size 6, 7, 8
- Laryngeal mask airway (LMA) size 3, 4, 5 (in case bag mask ventilation is impossible, as a backup)

Technique (Figure 15.2)
This may be tolerated in an awake or semi-conscious patient who will not tolerate an oropharyngeal airway. It is also useful when mouth opening is reduced. **It is contraindicated in patients with basal skull fracture.**

1. Size the airway. Place the wide phalange level with the chosen nostril, the bevelled end should reach the tragus.
2. Check the airway has a patent lumen. Some come with a safety pin – if so this should be pinned through the phalange (Figure 15.2b) before use of the airway on the patient.
3. Ask the patient if they have a better nostril for breathing through or one side that is blocked. Choose the most patent nostril for airway insertion (often the right).
4. Stand at the head end of the patient. Inform the patient that you will introduce the airway into the chosen nostril.
5. Lightly lubricate the outer surface of the airway (take care not to get too much lubrication on your gloves as it becomes difficult to manipulate the airway).
6. Introduce the airway with the 'sharp' end of the bevel adjacent to the medial wall of the nose (to avoid traumatising the turbinates).
7. Advance the airway perpendicular to the floor of the nose. You should not be aiming caudate, as you risk traumatising the narrow cribriform plate that separates the nasal cavity from the anterior cranial fossa. Aim directly in line with the tragus (see Figure 15.3).

Aftercare
1. Place the sedated or unconscious patient in the recovery position so that the airway can be easily cleared if the patient regurgitates or vomits.
2. If the patient starts to cough or choke remove the airway.
3. Ensure the patient is accompanied by a trained person to monitor for continued airway patency until (i) they regain consciousness (if sedated or post seizure), or (ii) help arrives to site a definitive airway.
4. Minimum monitoring includes oxygen saturation (SaO_2), respiratory rate, and looking, listening, and feeling for airway patency.
5. Remove the airway gently and check for blood on the outer surface. Be prepared for bleeding into the airway.

Common anatomical pitfalls
1. Failing to follow the floor of the nose when siting a nasopharyngeal airway can traumatise the middle turbinate.
2. The turbinates are bone folds covered in respiratory mucosa. The inferior turbinate is the largest and can be a vascular structure, especially in a patient with nasal congestion or polyps. Trauma to the turbinates can cause early epistaxis or late rhinitis.
3. Little's area is a section of exposed mucosa found in the anterior part of the nasal cavity. It gains its blood supply from Kiesselbach's plexus, an anastomosis of the sphenopalatine artery (a continuation of the maxillary artery), the superior labial and ascending branch of the greater palatine artery. Trauma to Little's area can cause severe epistaxis.
4. The narrowest part of the airway is along the floor of the nose just before the change from nasal cavity to nasopharynx. Rotating the airway counterclockwise with gentle forward pressure can help to pass the airway.
5. Septal deviation is common and can occur anteriorly in the cartilaginous septum, or less frequently posteriorly in the bony septum. A patient with long-standing deviation of the septum may have contralateral hypertrophy of the inferior turbinate resulting in bilateral narrowed nasal passage.

Top tips
1. Nasopharyngeal airway sizing – mostly size 6 for small adult females, size 7 for females, size for 7 males, and size 8 for large males.
2. If in doubt, choose a nasopharyngeal airway with an outer diameter the same thickness as the patient's little finger.
3. A history of bad snoring should alert you to potential airway collapse and obstruction in a sedated patient.
4. Nasopharyngeal airways are better tolerated in the awake patient with respiratory distress. They also permit the passage of a soft suction catheter to facilitate naso- and oropharyngeal toilet.
5. On average it is 12 cm from the teeth to the larynx in women and 14 cm in men.

16 Laryngeal mask airway

Jane Sturgess

Figure 16.1 Different LMAs.

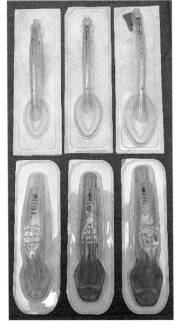

Figure 16.2 Patient position for insertion of LMA (plus sagittal anatomy).

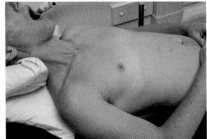

Figure 16.3 How to hold the LMA.

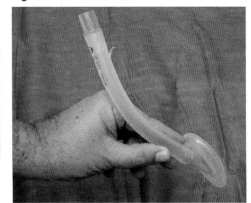

Figure 16.4 Anatomical position of a correctly positioned LMA.

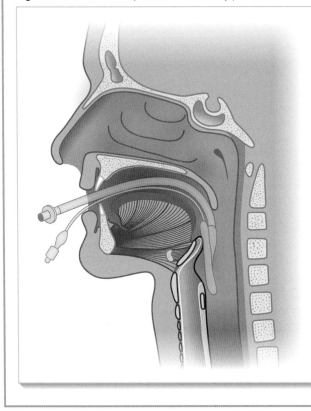

Figure 16.5 Soft tissue trauma following poorly inserted LMA. Reproduced with permission from Reid et al., published in The Laryngoscope © 2019 The American Laryngological, Rhinological and Otological Society, Inc.

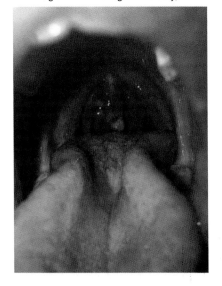

Applied Anatomy for Clinical Procedures at a Glance, First Edition. Jane Sturgess, Francesca Crawley, Ramez Kirollos, and Kirsty Cattle.
© 2021 John Wiley & Sons Ltd. Published 2021 by John Wiley & Sons Ltd.

Equipment

As airway adjuncts (Chapter 15)

- Laryngeal mask airway (LMA) size 3 or 4 ♀, or 4 or 5 ♂ (Figure 16.1)
- 20 mL syringe filled with air, and spare syringe
- Lubricating jelly
- Tape to secure the LMA

Technique

This should only ever be performed under direct supervision (by an experienced practitioner). Patients with cervical spine injury are not suitable candidates for the inexperienced.

1. Check the lumen of the LMA is patent. Inflate the cuff to check its integrity, then deflate it. NB. Cuff volumes size 3 = 20 mL, size 4 = 30 mL, size 5 = 40 mL.
2. Lightly lubricate the convex surface of the elliptical end of the LMA taking care not to deposit a blob of gel over/in the glottic aperture.
3. Monitor the oxygen saturation (SaO_2), blood pressure, and electrocardiogram.
4. Pre-oxygenate the patient (15 l/min O_2 via a tight fitting mask) either for 3 minutes or with 3 vital capacity breaths.
5. In the non-arrested patient an anaesthetic will be required.
6. When anaesthetised place the head in the 'sniffing the morning air' position, with the neck flexed and the head extended (Figure 16.2).
7. Open the mouth with your left hand and hold the LMA in your right hand.
8. Hold the LMA like it is a pencil with the tip of your index finger sitting in the dimple between the elliptical cuff and the tube (Figure 16.3). The aperture should be facing uppermost so that it will follow the tongue and sit (open) over the laryngeal inlet.
9. Use your finger to guide the convex side of the cuff along the midline of the hard palate, through the mouth into the oropharynx, before being advanced into the hypopharynx.
10. Your finger should stay in the dimple until you feel it at the posterior border of the tongue. At this point hold the proximal end of the tube between your left index finger and thumb and advance the tube into the hypopharynx (Figure 16.4).
11. You will feel a 'stop'.
12. Keep hold of your inserted LMA and inflate the cuff.
13. Attach the 15 mm connector to a breathing circuit or Ambu Bag and gently insufflate to check that the chest rises and falls with each breath and that CO_2 is detected by the capnograph.
14. Secure your LMA in place.

Aftercare

1. The patency of the airway and the position of the LMA should be regularly checked whilst it remains in situ. Watching the chest rise and fall, whilst the breathing is quiet, and CO_2 is detected by the capnograph, can often do this.
2. LMAs can cause stimulation of the airway and result in bronchospasm. This is an emergency and requires experienced help to manage it. If you think you may have caused this remove the LMA and resume bag mask ventilation.

Common anatomical pitfalls

1. The LMA is designed to sit in the patient's hypopharynx and cover the supraglottic structures, thereby allowing relative isolation of the trachea. If the device is turned during its insertion the airway will be partially occluded, and the trachea less isolated and at greater risk if the patients regurgitates stomach contents.
2. Tongue ulceration can be caused if the tongue is trapped between the LMA and the teeth, when tissue pressure exceeds intracapillary pressure in the lingual artery (a branch of the external carotid).
3. Ulceration and/or necrosis of the uvula occurs by compression of soft tissue between the hard palate and the LMA with tissue pressure exceeding intracapillary pressure of ascending palatine artery (a branch of the facial artery) (Figure 16.5).
4. Lingual nerve damage (a branch of the third division of the trigeminal nerve) causing numbness or dysaesthesia can be caused by direct trauma as the tongue is manipulated during LMA insertion, or by compression of blood supply (as in 2 and 3) to the nerve, resulting in nerve injury.

Top tips

1. The widest part of the LMA is at the junction of the cuff and the tube. If the patient has reduced mouth opening this can be the most difficult part to advance into the mouth. Remove your finger and ask an assistant to perform a jaw thrust. Once in the mouth (and past the teeth) resume your standard technique.
2. Keeping your finger in the dimple and guiding the LMA along the hard palate will stop the LMA tip folding back on itself.
3. If the tip continually folds back, first try deflating the cuff completely. If this does not help, try inflating the cuff with 10 mL of air.
4. In patients that obstruct their airway with a large tongue, or a small jaw, a jaw thrust can help you pass the LMA from the mouth into the oropharynx, and on into the hypopharynx (i.e. it opens the airway to better allow you to 'turn the corner'.)
5. If you have any concern of regurgitation or aspiration an endotracheal tube is the device of choice. In the emergency a patent airway is the priority. If you are having difficulty maintaining a patent airway with bag mask ventilation, choose a supraglottic airway with an accessory port that will permit suction or the passage of a nasogastric tube.

17 Central venous cannulation (high approach internal jugular)

Jane Sturgess

Figure 17.1 Equipment required.

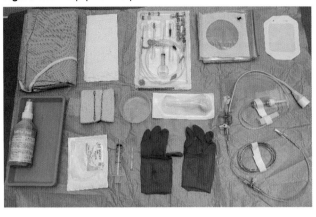

Figure 17.2 Patient positioning.

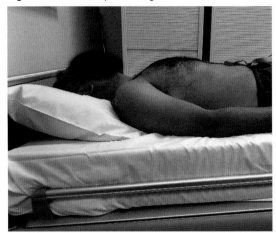

Figure 17.3 Procedure – see text for explanation.

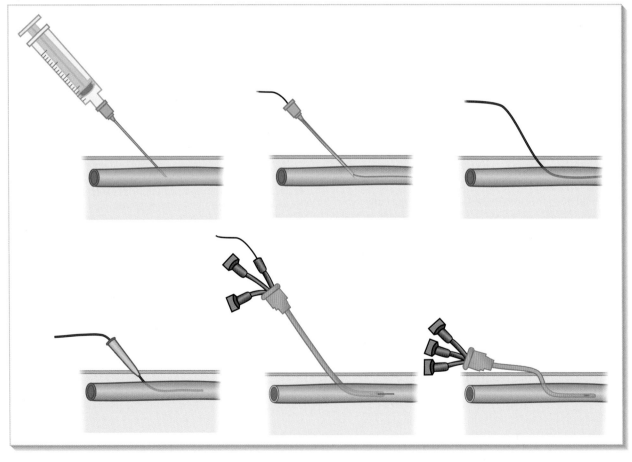

Applied Anatomy for Clinical Procedures at a Glance, First Edition. Jane Sturgess, Francesca Crawley, Ramez Kirollos, and Kirsty Cattle.

Figure 17.4 Internal jugular landmarks.

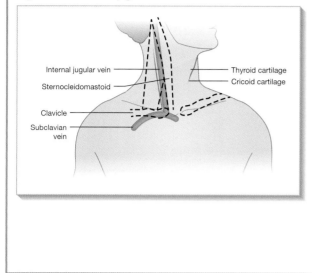

Figure 17.5 Chest X-ray showing central venous catheter in correct position.

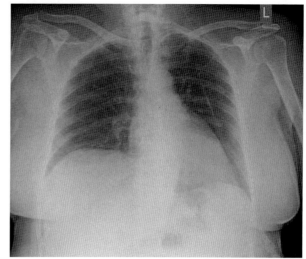

How to insert a central venous line

Prior to starting, assess patient for contraindications:
- Uncooperative patient
- Abnormal clotting
- Haemo- or pneumothorax on contralateral side
- Only one functioning lung
- Infection over puncture site

Equipment (Figure 17.1)

Central line kit comprising:
- Venous catheter (generally 20 cm long, use catheter which is 15 cm long if performing right neck catheterisation)
- Guidewire in plastic sheath
- Guide syringe and needle
- 'Big' needle
- Anaesthetising syringe and needle
- Sponge for putting needles and syringes in
- Lignocaine
- Scalpel
- Drapes, gauzes, suturing needle

In addition:
- Full sterile kit (gown, gloves, hat, sterile sheath for ultrasound probe)
- Ultrasound for guidance

Technique (Figure 17.3)

Identify patient and assemble equipment.
1. Check it is the correct patient by asking them to state their name.
2. Obtain patient consent.
3. Place patient in Trendelenburg position (feet up, head down to increase venous pressure, see Figure 17.2).
4. Establish which vein you will cannulate.
5. Identify landmarks (see right column) and use ultrasound to identify vein.
6. Wash hands, open pack, and apply sterile gloves.
7. Clean skin using disinfectant and drape area.
8. Fill wells in kit with saline.
9. Flush ports of line with saline (to ensure all are patent).
10. Attach clips to each line (to be used later to 'close' each port).
11. Use 'big' needle initially (the guidewire will only fit through this needle).
12. Attach 'big' needle to syringe with bevel aligned with the numbers on the syringe.
13. Place three syringes in order: small for anaesthesia, medium for finding vein, large for placing guidewire.
14. Use lignocaine to anesthetise venepuncture area and suture area.
15. Use either medium or big needle and advance needle using negative pressure until flashback of blood seen. Change to big needle if currently using medium.
16. Feed guidewire through big needle and into vein (Seldinger technique). Should go easily. If not, rotate it or withdraw a little and retry.
17. Withdraw needle, holding onto guidewire at all times.
18. Using a twisting movement, pass dilator over guidewire until it reaches the skin.
19. Take dilator out, using gauze to stop any bleeding.
20. Insert catheter over guidewire. The end of the guidewire should extend through the brown port.
21. Keep holding guidewire and insert catheter into vein until double line is reached.
22. Aspirate blood from brown port and then flush with saline.
23. Repeat for other two ports.
24. Suture catheter to skin. Use two openings on each side of the catheter hub.

Landmarks for internal jugular vein (Figure 17.4)

1. Locate the posterior border of sternomastoid, at the level of the cricoid cartilage.
2. Direct the needle towards the ipsilateral nipple (or towards the vein if ultrasound is being used – you will see how close the vein and artery lie).
3. Advance needle and aspirate. (Blood should be aspirated within 2 cm.)
4. When you aspirate blood, advance needle a little to check you are in the vein.

The internal jugular vein in the neck lies within the carotid sheath, lateral to the carotid artery together with the common carotid artery and vagus. This lies on the scalenus anterior muscle with the sympathetic trunk which is outside the carotid sheath and lies deeper to it on that muscle.

The internal jugular vein passes from the carotid triangle (part of the anterior triangle of the neck) – between the medial border of the sternomastoid, the posterior belly of the digastric, and the superior belly of the omohyoid – deep to the sternomastoid and joins the subclavian vein in the subclavian triangle (part of the posterior triangle of the neck) – between the sternomastoid, superior border of the clavicle and the inferior belly of the omohyoid – deep to the sternomastoid.

Aftercare

1. Arrange a chest X-ray to ensure the line is in the correct place (Figure 17.5) and to exclude a pneumothorax. The apex of the pleura extends about 3–4 cm superior to the sternal end of the first rib in proximity to the subclavian vessels.

2. Document procedure.

Common complications

- Pneumothorax
- Haematoma
- Arterial puncture
- Haemorrhage
- Air emboli
- Cardiac arrhythmias

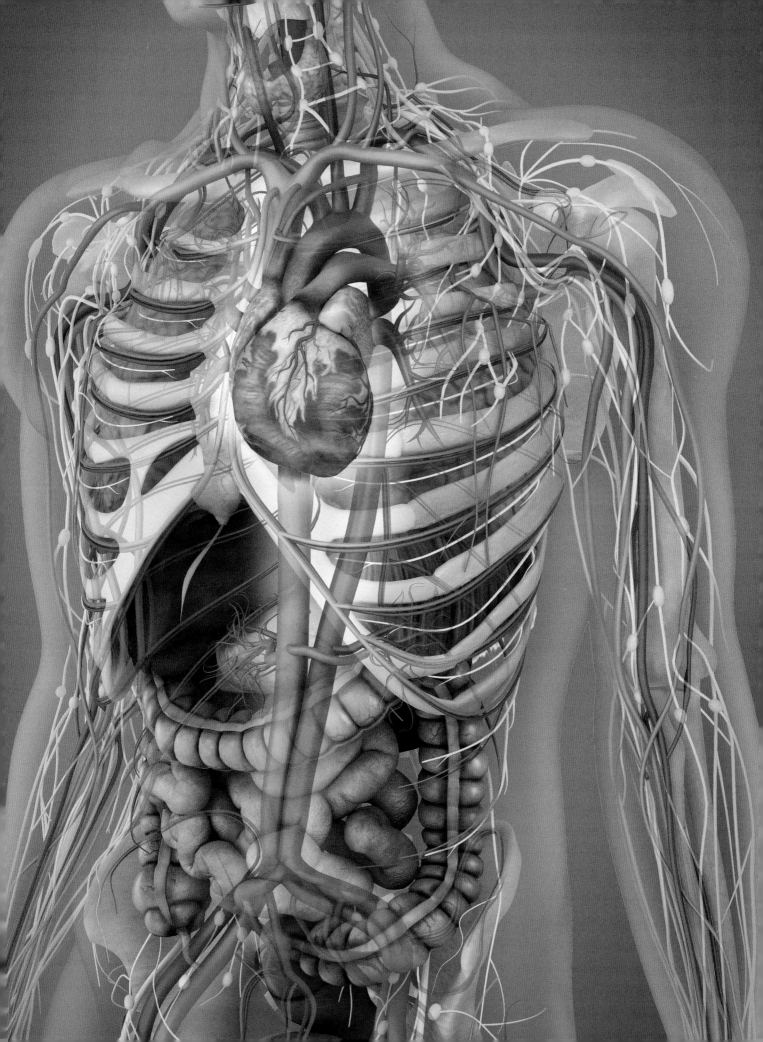

18 Central venous cannulation (low approach internal jugular)

Jane Sturgess

Figure 18.1 Equipment required.

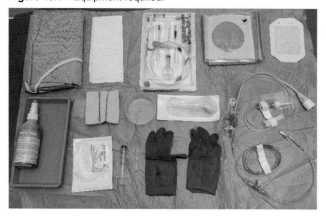

Figure 18.2 Patient positioning.

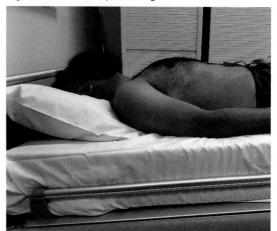

Figure 18.3 Procedure.

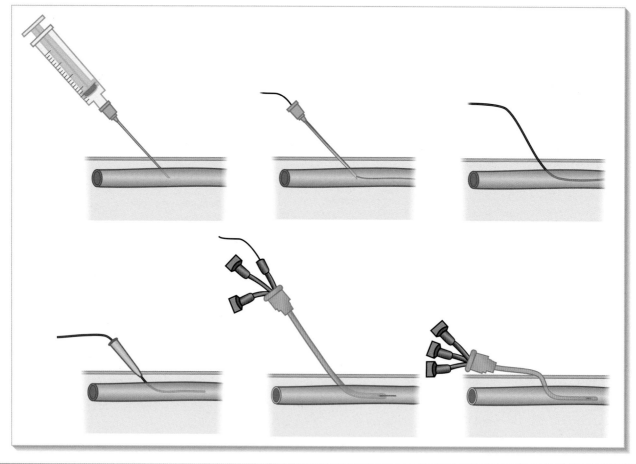

Applied Anatomy for Clinical Procedures at a Glance, First Edition. Jane Sturgess, Francesca Crawley, Ramez Kirollos, and Kirsty Cattle.

Figure 18.4 Internal jugular landmarks.

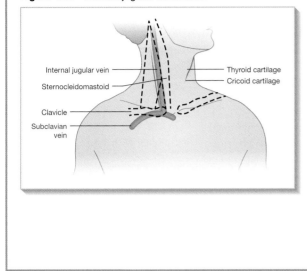

Figure 18.5 Chest X-ray showing central venous catheter in correct position.

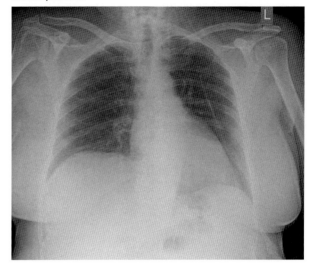

How to insert a central venous line

Prior to starting, assess patient for contraindications:

- Uncooperative patient
- Abnormal clotting
- Haemo or pneumothorax on contralateral side
- Only one functioning lung
- Infection over puncture site

Equipment (Figure 18.1)

Central line kit comprising:

- Venous catheter (generally 20 cm long, use catheter which is 15 cm long if performing right neck catheterisation)
- Guidewire in plastic sheath
- Guide syringe and needle
- 'Big' needle
- Anaesthetising syringe and needle
- Sponge for putting needles and syringes in
- Lignocaine
- Scalpel
- Drapes, gauzes, suturing needle

In addition:

- Full sterile kit (gown, gloves, hat, sterile sheath for ultrasound probe)
- Ultrasound for guidance

Technique (Figure 18.3)

Identify patient and assemble equipment.

1. Check it is the correct patient by asking them to state their name.
2. Obtain patient consent.
3. Place patient in Trendelenburg position (feet up, head down to increase venous pressure, see Figure 18.2).
4. Establish which vein you will cannulate.
5. Identify landmarks (see right column) and use ultrasound to identify vein.
6. Wash hands, open pack, and apply sterile gloves.
7. Clean skin using disinfectant and drape area.
8. Fill wells in kit with saline.
9. Flush ports of line with saline (to ensure all are patent).
10. Attach clips to each line (to be used later to 'close' each port).
11. Use 'big' needle initially (the guidewire will only fit through this needle).
12. Attach 'big' needle to syringe with bevel aligned with the numbers on the syringe.
13. Place three syringes in order: small for anaesthesia, medium for finding vein, large for placing guidewire.
14. Use lignocaine to anesthetise venepuncture area and suture area.
15. Use either medium or big needle and advance needle using negative pressure until flashback of blood seen. Change to big needle if currently using medium.
16. Feed guidewire through big needle and into vein (Seldinger technique). Should go easily. If not, rotate it or withdraw a little and retry.
17. Withdraw needle, holding onto guidewire at all times.
18. Using a twisting movement, pass dilator over guidewire until it reaches the skin.
19. Take dilator out, using gauze to stop any bleeding.
20. Insert catheter over guidewire. The end of the guidewire should extend through the brown port.
21. Keep holding guidewire and insert catheter into vein until double line is reached.
22. Aspirate blood from brown port and then flush with saline.
23. Repeat for other two ports.
24. Suture catheter to skin. Use two openings on each side of the catheter hub.

Landmarks for internal jugular vein (Figure 18.4)

1. Identify a triangle in the neck formed by the two heads of sternocleidomastoid.
2. Penetrate the skin at the apex of the triangle: needle at 30 degrees to skin.
3. Aim at ipsilateral nipple.
4. Advance needle and aspirate.
5. When you aspirate blood, advance needle a little to check you are in the vein.

The internal jugular vein in the neck lies within the carotid sheath, lateral to the carotid artery together with the common carotid artery and vagus. This lies on the scalenus anterior muscle with the sympathetic trunk which is outside the carotid sheath and lies deeper to it on that muscle.

The internal jugular vein passes from the carotid triangle (part of the anterior triangle of the neck) – between the medial border of the sternomastoid, the posterior belly of the digastric, and the superior belly of the omohyoid – deep to the sternomastoid and joins the subclavian vein in the subclavian triangle (part of the posterior triangle of the neck) – between the sternomastoid, superior border of the clavicle and the inferior belly of the omohyoid – deep to the sternomastoid.

Aftercare

1. Arrange a chest X-ray to ensure the line is in the correct place (Figure 18.5) and to exclude a pneumothorax. The apex of the pleura extends about 3–4 cm superior to the sternal end of the first rib in proximity to the subclavian vessels.
2. Document procedure.

Common complications

- Pneumothorax – higher with low approach
- Haematoma
- Arterial puncture
- Haemorrhage
- Air emboli
- Cardiac arrhythmias
- Punctured ventricle – risk higher with low approach (need shorter length of line)

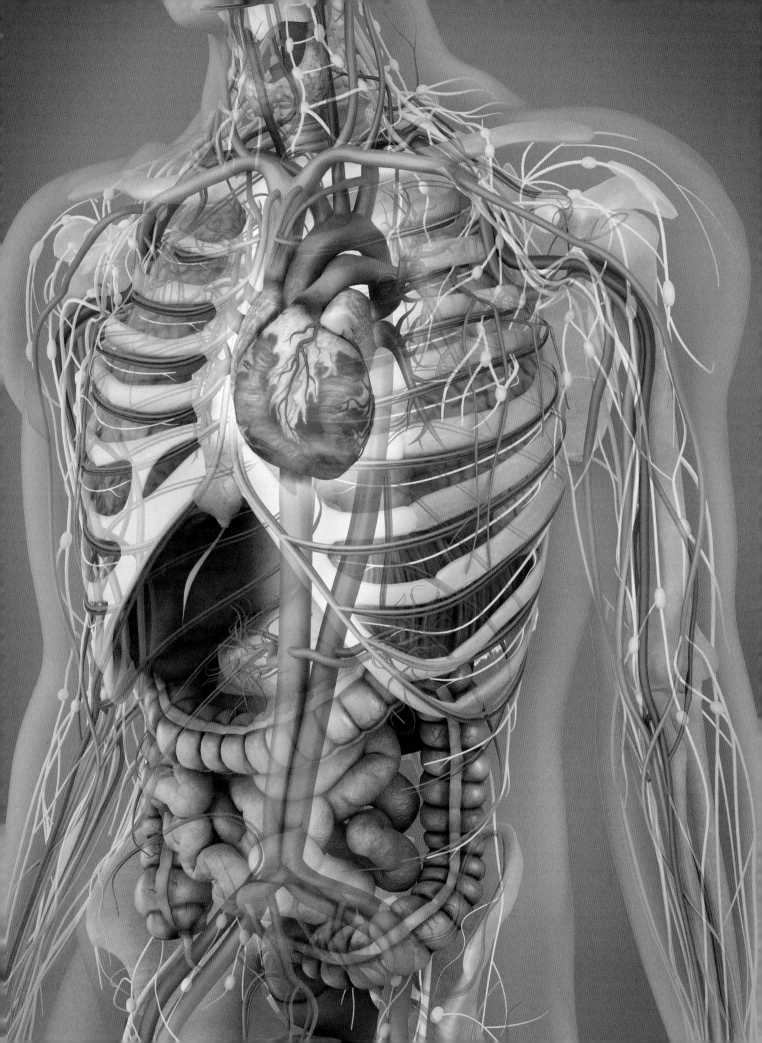

19 Central venous cannulation (subclavian)

Jane Sturgess

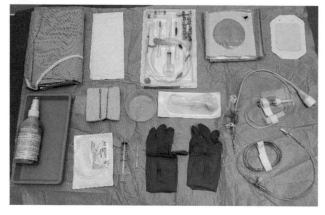

Figure 19.1 Equipment required.

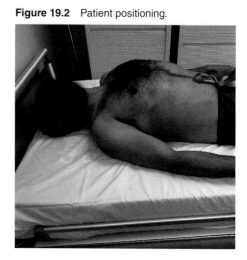

Figure 19.2 Patient positioning.

Figure 19.3 Procedure.

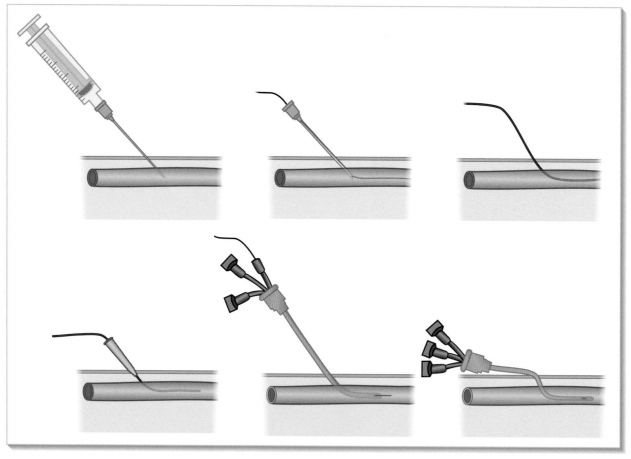

Applied Anatomy for Clinical Procedures at a Glance, First Edition. Jane Sturgess, Francesca Crawley, Ramez Kirollos, and Kirsty Cattle.
© 2021 John Wiley & Sons Ltd. Published 2021 by John Wiley & Sons Ltd.

Figure 19.4 Subclavian vein landmarks.

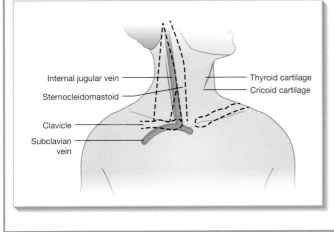

Figure 19.5 Chest X-ray showing central venous catheter in correct position.

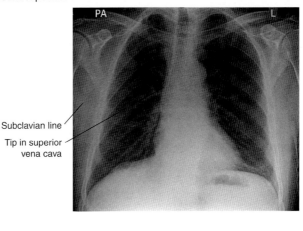

How to insert a central venous line

Prior to starting, assess patient for contraindications:

- Uncooperative patient
- Abnormal clotting
- Haemo- or pneumothorax on contralateral side
- Only one functioning lung
- Infection over puncture site

Equipment (Figure 19.1)

Central line kit comprising:

- Venous catheter (generally 20 cm long, use catheter which is 15 cm long if performing right neck catheterisation)
- Guidewire in plastic sheath
- Guide syringe and needle
- 'Big' needle
- Anaesthetising syringe and needle
- Sponge for putting needles and syringes in
- Lignocaine
- Scalpel
- Drapes, gauzes, suturing needle

In addition:

- Full sterile kit (gown, gloves, hat, sterile sheath for ultrasound probe)
- Ultrasound for guidance

Technique (Figure 19.3)

Identify patient and assemble equipment.

1. Check it is the correct patient by asking them to state their name.
2. Obtain patient consent.
3. Place patient in Trendelenburg position (feet up, head down to increase venous pressure; see Figure 19.2).
4. Establish which vein you will cannulate.
5. Identify landmarks (see right column) and use ultrasound to identify vein.
6. Wash hands, open pack, and apply sterile gloves.
7. Clean skin using disinfectant and drape area.
8. Fill wells in kit with saline.
9. Flush ports. of line with saline (to ensure all are patent)
10. Attach clips to each line (to be used later to 'close' each port).

11. Use 'big' needle initially (the guidewire will only fit through this needle).
12. Attach 'big' needle to syringe with bevel aligned with the numbers on the syringe.
13. Place three syringes in order: small for anaesthesia, medium for finding vein, large for placing guidewire.
14. Use lignocaine to anesthetise venepuncture area and suture area.
15. Use either medium or big needle and advance needle using negative pressure until flashback of blood seen. Change to big needle if currently using medium.
16. Feed guidewire through big needle and into vein (Seldinger technique). Should go easily. If not, rotate it or withdraw a little and retry.
17. Withdraw needle, holding onto guidewire at all times.
18. Using a twisting movement, pass dilator over guidewire until it reaches the skin.
19. Take dilator out, using gauze to stop any bleeding.
20. Insert catheter over guidewire. The end of the guidewire should extend through the brown port.
21. Keep holding guidewire and insert catheter into vein until double line is reached.
22. Aspirate blood from brown port and then flush with saline.
23. Repeat for other two ports.
24. Suture catheter to skin. Use two openings on each side of the catheter hub.

Aftercare

1. Arrange a chest X-ray to ensure the line is in the correct place (Figure 19.5) and to exclude a pneumothorax. The apex of the pleura extends about 3–4 cm superior to the sternal end of the first rib in proximity to the subclavian vessels.
2. Document procedure.

Common complications

- Pneumothorax
- Haematoma
- Arterial puncture
- Haemorrhage
- Air emboli
- Cardiac arrhythmias

Landmarks for subclavian vein (Figure 19.4)

1. One centimetre lateral to the junction of the medial and middle third of the clavicle
2. Introduce the needle a finger-breadth below the clavicle and, whilst aspirating, advance towards the suprasternal notch under and along the inferior border of the clavicle until the vein is entered and blood is freely aspirated.
3. The subclavian vein course is deep to the clavicle and is hardly above the level of its upper border with omohyoid superiorly and the subclavius muscle inferiorly deep to the clavicle are lying superficial to the plane of the vein. It is separated from the deeply located second part of the subclavian artery by the scalenus anterior muscle. At the medial border of the scalenus anterior muscle the subclavian vein joins the internal jugular vein to form the brachiocephalic vein.

Top tips

- Place a bag of 500 mL bag of saline longitudinally between scapulae – it opens the chest wall.
- If still difficult, pull shoulder down and supinate the hand to open up the infraclavicular space.
- Keep the needle superficial. The artery lies deep to the vein and if you hit it, it is inaccessible for compression.

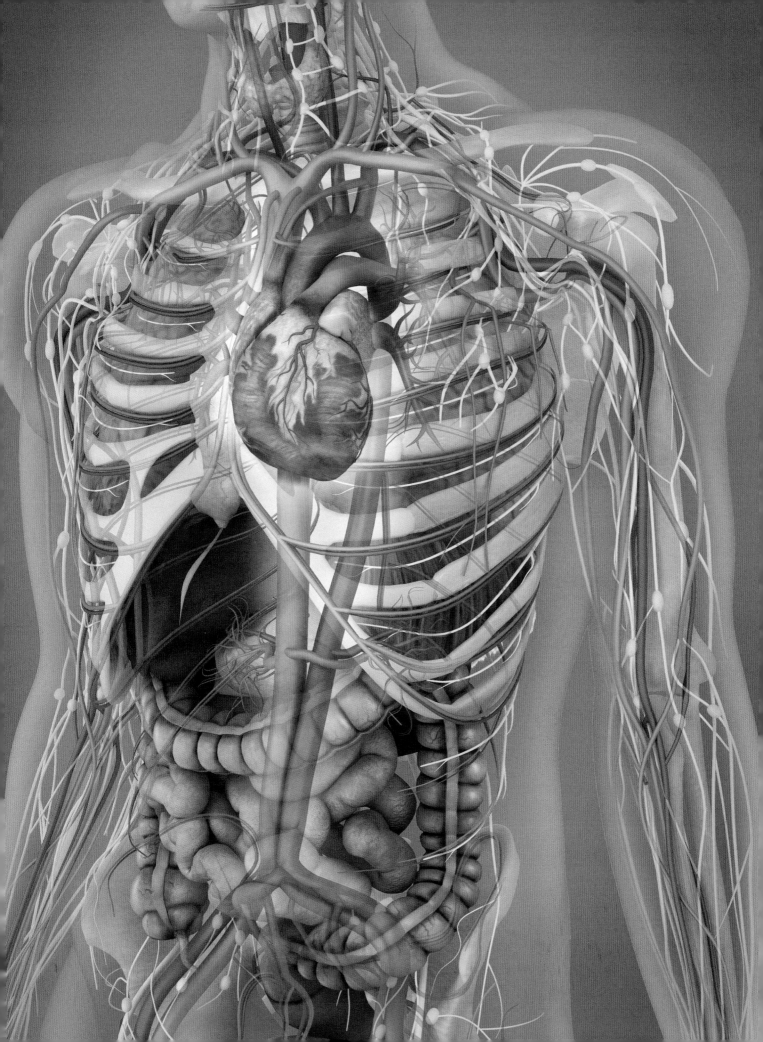

20 Direct current cardioversion

Francesca Crawley

Figure 20.1 Equipment.

Figure 20.2 Patient position.

Figure 20.3 Lead position.

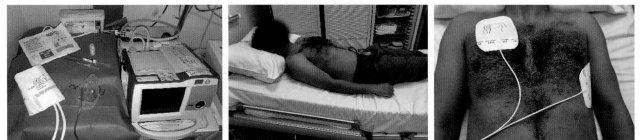

Figure 20.4 Synchronising the cardioverter.

Figure 20.5 Charging the cardioverter.

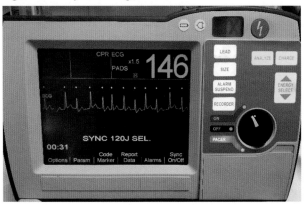

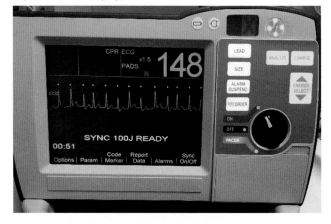

Figure 20.6 ECG pre DC cardioversion.

Figure 20.7 ECG post successful DC cardioversion.

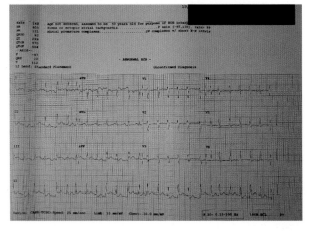

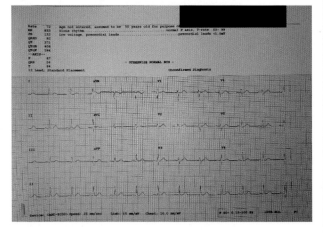

Applied Anatomy for Clinical Procedures at a Glance, First Edition. Jane Sturgess, Francesca Crawley, Ramez Kirollos, and Kirsty Cattle.
© 2021 John Wiley & Sons Ltd. Published 2021 by John Wiley & Sons Ltd.

How to perform direct current (DC) cardioversion:

Indications

DC cardioversion is used to convert atrial fibrillation, atrial flutter, atrial tachycardia, and supraventricular tachycardia to sinus rhythm.

Equipment (Figure 20.1)

- DC cardioverter
- Cannula (19 gauge) and equipment to insert it
- Short acting intravenous sedative drug (generally midazolam, 2–3 mg; check local policy)
- Razor to shave excessive chest hair (for pad contact)
- DC cardioversion pads
- Oxygen supply and mask
- Blood pressure cuff and automated monitor

Contraindications

- Pulseless ventricular tachycardia and fibrillation – these patients require advanced life support and a cardiac arrest call.

Pre-procedure

1. Check patient's details, explain the procedure, and obtain consent.
2. Lay patient at 30 degrees with their head on a pillow (Figure 20.2).
3. Perform an electrocardiogram (ECG) to confirm that the patient is in an appropriate rhythm (Figure 20.6).
4. Sedate patient with intravenous drug (generally midazolam).
5. Attach the leads from the cardioverter to the patient's limbs (as the limb ECG leads) and confirm the heart rhythm is showing on the monitor.
6. Inspect right upper chest for hair. The pad needs to make good skin contact and excessive hair may need to be shaved.
7. Attach DC cardioversion pads, one to left flank (Figure 20.3) and one over right upper chest (anterolateral position).
8. Attach leads from pads to the monitor.
9. Confirm rhythm on the monitor.

Procedure

1. Press the 'synchronisation' button on the monitor and check the 'synchronising' light is on (Figure 20.4). Observe the monitor for little triangles marking the tops of the R waves. This indicates that the machine is synchronising correctly.

2. Select energy setting on the monitor. For a broad-complex tachycardia or atrial fibrillation, start with 120–150 Joules and increase in increments if this fails. For atrial flutter and regular narrow complex tachycardia, start with 70–120 Joules (Resuscitation Council guidelines, 2015, available at https://www.resus.org.uk/resuscitation-guidelines; will be updated in 2020).
3. Explain to the patient that you are about to attempt cardioversion and that it may be uncomfortable.
4. Press the 'print' button on the monitor (so you have a record of the rhythm pre and post attempted DC cardioversion).
5. Verbally clear the area, ensuring no member of the team is touching the bed or patient.
6. Press 'charge' on the monitor.
7. Watch charge screen fill, indicating that the machine is charged (Figure 20.5).
8. Press 'discharge' button on monitor and hold the button until the machine 'clicks', indicating that energy has been delivered.
9. Recheck the monitor. If the patient is back in sinus rhythm, move to the post procedure steps, otherwise return to step 1. Establish what shock you should now attempt (generally 100 Joules).

Post-procedure

1. Check the patient is OK and measure their pulse rate and blood pressure.
2. Perform a 12 lead ECG to confirm sinus rhythm (Figure 20.7).
3. Continue to monitor the patient's blood pressure and pulse for 30 minutes.

Top tip

- Select lead II for monitoring purposes, as this is the best lead for identifying a P wave after the procedure and confirming sinus rhythm.

Pitfalls

- Ensure the 'synchronisation' button is pressed and that the light is on. Failure to do this could result in shocking the patient into ventricular fibrillation, if the shock is delivered on the T-wave (repolarisation).
- If the synchronisation light is on but the triangles are not visible, try changing the lead that the monitor is displaying. There is a dial on the monitor for this.

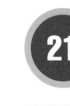

21 Intercostal drains

Francesca Crawley

Figure 21.1 Equipment.

Figure 21.2 Patient positioning and "window of safety", bordered by pectoralis major anteriorly, latissimus dorsi posteriorly, the fifth intercostal space inferiorly, and the base of the axilla superiorly.

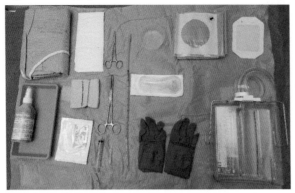

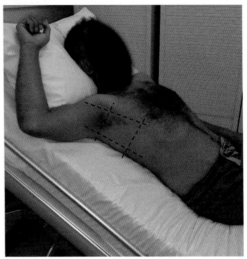

Figure 21.3 Thoracic anatomy. Note the position of the neurovascular bundle in relation to the rib.

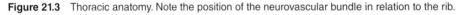

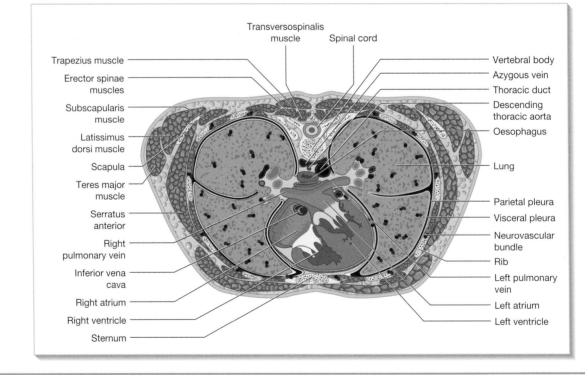

Trapezius muscle
Erector spinae muscles
Subscapularis muscle
Latissimus dorsi muscle
Scapula
Teres major muscle
Serratus anterior
Right pulmonary vein
Inferior vena cava
Right atrium
Right ventricle
Sternum

Transversospinalis muscle
Spinal cord

Vertebral body
Azygous vein
Thoracic duct
Descending thoracic aorta
Oesophagus

Lung

Parietal pleura
Visceral pleura
Neurovascular bundle
Rib
Left pulmonary vein
Left atrium
Left ventricle

Applied Anatomy for Clinical Procedures at a Glance, First Edition. Jane Sturgess, Francesca Crawley, Ramez Kirollos, and Kirsty Cattle.
© 2021 John Wiley & Sons Ltd. Published 2021 by John Wiley & Sons Ltd.

Requirements
- Written consent (see Chapter 6)
- Clean area to perform procedure
- Experienced operator (or supervisor)
- Nursing staff familiar with chest drains
- Recent chest X-ray

Equipment (Figure 21.1)
- Sterile pack containing gloves, gown, mask, two drapes
- Underwater sealed drain system, with valve mechanism to prevent air or fluid entering pleural cavity (see Chapter 9)
- Intercostal drain:
  - Small bore (Seldinger) for small pneumothorax or effusion
  - Non-Seldinger (large bore) for large pneumothorax, haemothorax, or empyema. These are generally inserted surgically.
- Antiseptic solution
- 20 mL 1% lignocaine
- 5 mL syringe and needle, gauze swabs
- Scalpel blade
- Suture material: 0 or 1-0 silk with needle
- Tape and dressing to secure tube to chest wall
- Oximetry and cardiac monitor

Procedure – Seldinger technique
If the drain is required for fluid, ultrasound guidance is strongly recommended.
1. Position conscious patient in sitting position at 45 degrees with arm of same side placed above head (Figure 21.2).
2. Palpate the fourth or fifth intercostal space in mid axillary line.
3. Clean and drape the area.
4. Infiltrate local anaesthetic into the skin, then aim to touch the superior aspect of the 5th rib and instil local anaesthetic to cover periosteal pain, advance the needle horizontally about 2 mm until you feel a 'pop' – this will be pleura – and instil local anaesthetic here.
5. Attempt to aspirate air or fluid with your local anaesthetic syringe and needle. If this is impossible, you may not have reached the intrapleural space, consider advancing the needle slowly and carefully whilst gently aspirating on the syringe. If you remain unsuccessful abandon the procedure.
6. Insert the Tuohy needle (supplied with the Seldinger kit) into the pleural space. Aim the bevel of the Tuohy needle upwards for pneumothoraces and downwards for effusions.
7. Advance the tip of the Tuohy needle through the pleura and aspirate air or fluid.
8. Withdraw the syringe and pass the wire through the needle. It should pass easily. The Touhy needle is 8 cm long and the wire has cm markers along it – the wire will need to be 10–15 cm at the hub of the Touhy needle for the wire to be within the pleural space.
9. Remove the needle over the wire.
10. Make a small nick in the skin to ease the passage of the dilator. Pass the dilator over the wire. Do not insert the dilator more than 1 cm beyond the skin.
11. Remove the dilator over the wire, avoiding pulling the wire out!
12. Place drain over wire. Insert to 12–16 cm.
13. Remove wire and inner tube from drain. Attach three-way tap and leave closed until drain is attached to drainage system.
14. Secure drain to skin with a suture, indenting drain slightly to ensure it stays in.
15. Apply a purpose designed dressing (e.g. 'Drainfix').
16. Connect drain to tubing and open three-way tap.
17. Check underwater seal oscillates during respiration.
18. Order repeat chest X-ray.
19. Prescribe regular analgesia.

Procedure – Surgical technique
Start as per steps 1–5 of the Seldinger technique.
1. Once air or fluid is found, make a 1.5–2 cm incision in skin parallel to upper border of the rib below the chosen intercostal space.
2. Use a haemostat to dissect through the intercostal muscles and into the pleural space – you will feel a 'pop' as you open the pleura.
3. Pass your finger along the track you have dissected into the pleural space to check for adhesions.
4. Without removing your finger, clamp the external end of the chest drain and pass the drain along the track beside your finger and into the pleural space, directing it upwards for pneumothoraces and downwards for haemothoraces.
5. Secure the drain to the skin with a suture, indenting the drain slightly to ensure it stays in.
6. Connect the drain to the underwater seal (see Chapter 9) and release the clamp.
7. Check underwater seal oscillates during respiration.
8. Order repeat chest X-ray.
9. Prescribe regular analgesia.

Anatomical (and other) pitfalls
- It is relatively easy to force the chest drain into major organs; be gentle and do not use the introducer.
- The intercostal nerve and vessels lie under the rib (Figure 21.3); avoid these by making an incision above a rib. These are arranged in order with the vein uppermost, the artery in the middle, and the nerve lowermost. However, these give collateral branches running also in the intercostal space.
- The three layers of muscles in the intercostal space from superficial to deep are external intercostal, internal intercostal, and innermost intercostal muscles. The intercostal vessels and nerves are between the middle and innermost muscle layers.
- The 'triangle of safety' for insertion of intercostal drains is bordered by pectoralis major anteriorly, latissimus dorsi posteriorly, the fifth intercostal space inferiorly, and the base of the axilla superiorly (see Figure 21.2).
- All drain holes need to be within the pleural cavity. If they are not, surgical emphysema may occur.
- The parietal pleura is innervated by somatic intercostal nerves and the visceral pleura by the vagus. This explains the occasional transient reflex bradycardia that occurs when the deep layer of the pleura is mechanically irritated by the tip of the chest drain.
- Ensure tubing is 2 cm submerged in the collection chamber and keep this system below the patient or water can enter the pleural cavity.
- Do not drain more than one litre of fluid and clamp the tube at this point or if the patient experiences pain or starts to cough.
- Avoid purse string suturing as this can leave an unpleasant scar.

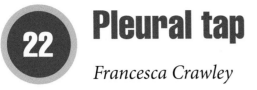

22 Pleural tap

Francesca Crawley

Figure 22.1 Equipment.

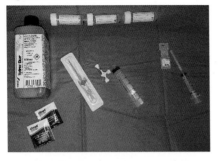

Figure 22.2 Patient positioning and 'window of safety'. Aspiration can be performed via the lumbar route or the 5th intercostal space.

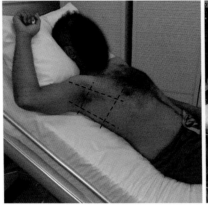
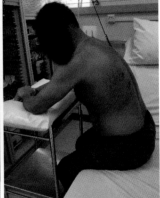

(a)   (b)

Figure 22.3 Connection of cannula to three-way tap and syringe with positions required.

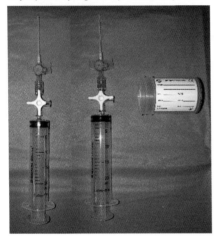

Figure 22.4 Thoracic anatomy. Note the position of the neurovascular bundle in relation to the rib.

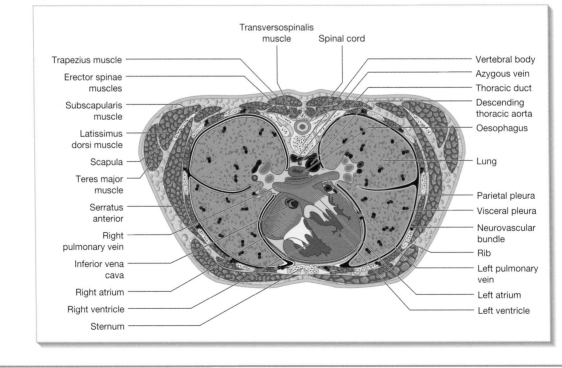

Transversospinalis muscle — Spinal cord

Trapezius muscle
Erector spinae muscles
Subscapularis muscle
Latissimus dorsi muscle
Scapula
Teres major muscle
Serratus anterior
Right pulmonary vein
Inferior vena cava
Right atrium
Right ventricle
Sternum

Vertebral body
Azygous vein
Thoracic duct
Descending thoracic aorta
Oesophagus
Lung
Parietal pleura
Visceral pleura
Neurovascular bundle
Rib
Left pulmonary vein
Left atrium
Left ventricle

Applied Anatomy for Clinical Procedures at a Glance, First Edition. Jane Sturgess, Francesca Crawley, Ramez Kirollos, and Kirsty Cattle.
© 2021 John Wiley & Sons Ltd. Published 2021 by John Wiley & Sons Ltd.

Requirements
- Verbal consent, cooperative patient
- Normal International Normalised Ratio (INR) (< 1.3) and platelet count > 50 × 10³/mL
- Recent chest X-ray
- Assistant
- Ultrasound-guided pre-marked aspiration site

Equipment (Figure 22.1)
- Large bore intravenous cannula
- Three-way tap
- 20 mL or 50 mL syringe
- Universal containers (×3)
- Disposal container
- Antiseptic skin cleanser
- Local anaesthetic, 18 or 20 gauge needle, 5 mL syringe

Procedure
If the drain is required for fluid, ultrasound guidance is strongly recommended. The British Thoracic Society recommends aspirating pleural fluid in the same manner as for insertion of an intercostal drain, via the window of safety above the 5th intercostal space. However, aspiration *can* be performed through the patient's back, where the pleural space extends more inferiorly.

1. Position the patient, preferably at 45 degrees with the arm of the same side placed above the head. However, if using the dorsal approach, sit the patient on the edge of his/her bed, leaning over a table, with pillow for support (Figure 22.2).
2. If the site of aspiration has not been marked with ultrasound guidance, determine the site of aspiration by percussion, comparing left and right. Confirm with the chest X-ray.
3. Surgically prepare the area.
4. Infiltrate the area with local anaesthetic (e.g. 5–10 mL 1% lignocaine), down to the pleura, going just over the top of the rib, to avoid the neurovascular bundle which runs just under the rib (Figure 22.4).
5. Insert the cannula into the pleural space.
6. Connect the cannula to the three-way tap and large syringe by removing the inner needle, leaving the plastic cannula in situ, being careful to avoid it kinking.
7. Close the three-way tap to air and open it to the patient and syringe.
8. Aspirate fluid.
9. Close the three-way tap to the patient and open it to the syringe and air (Figure 22.3).
10. Have an assistant hold a universal container beneath the open three-way tap and expel fluid into the universal container.
11. Close the three-way tap to air and open to the cannula and syringe.
12. Repeat steps 7 to 10 twice more, thus filling three universal containers.
13. Check the volume to be removed for therapeutic reasons.
14. Remove the cannula, apply gentle pressure for a short period, then apply a dressing.
15. Label and send the specimens to the laboratory, usually for (i) microbiology, (ii) cytology, and (iii) biochemistry for protein levels.
16. Thank the patient and ensure he/she is comfortable.

Anatomical (and other) pitfalls
- Inability to aspirate fluid. Examine the patient carefully before commencing to ensure your needle is likely to enter fluid. If unable to aspirate fluid, ask for repeat attempts under radiological guidance.
- In the anatomical position, the scapula extends as low as the seventh spinous process. It can be retracted forwards if the patient leans his/her arms forwards (as in Figure 22.2b) and out of the aspiration area.
- The pleural space extends inferiorly as far as T12, but the diaphragm (and underlying liver) rises as high as T10. Take care then not to insert the needle beyond the pleural space into the diaphragm or liver. Continuous aspiration while advancing the needle guards against this.

Complications
- Pneumothorax
- Procedure failure
- Pain
- Haemorrhage
- Visceral injury

23 Inserting a nasogastric tube

Francesca Crawley

Figure 23.1 Equipment.

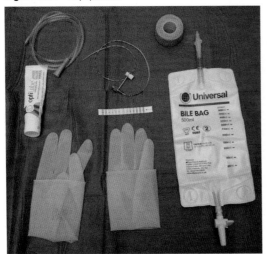

Figure 23.2 Different NG types.

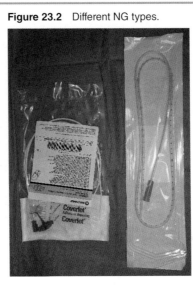

Figure 23.3 Patient position.

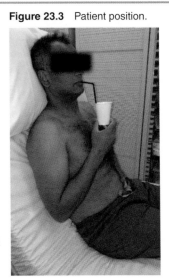

Figure 23.4 Estimate the length of insertion by holding the nasogastric tube (NGT) from the tip of the nose to the earlobe and then the xiphisternum.

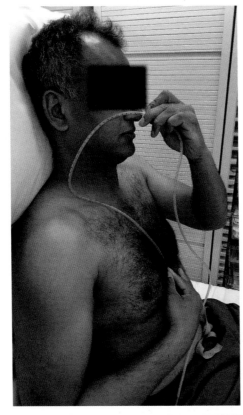

Figure 23.5 Chest X-ray showing NGT in correct position, tip going below diaphragm. Note this chest X-ray also shows central line and ECG monitoring lines.

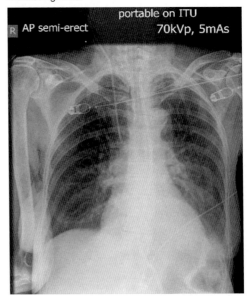

Applied Anatomy for Clinical Procedures at a Glance, First Edition. Jane Sturgess, Francesca Crawley, Ramez Kirollos, and Kirsty Cattle.
© 2021 John Wiley & Sons Ltd. Published 2021 by John Wiley & Sons Ltd.

How to insert a nasogastric tube (NGT):

Equipment (Figure 23.1)

- Non-sterile gloves
- Fine bore NGT (for feeding, contains guidewire) or nasogastric 'Ryles' tube (for draining stomach contents, no guidewire). See Figure 23.2.
- Lubricant (water based)
- Syringe
- Bile bag (if NGT is for drainage)
- Tape to secure NGT to skin
- Glass of water (and 'bendy' straw if preferred)
- pH paper

Procedure

1. Identify patient and assemble equipment.
2. Check it is the correct patient by asking them to state their name.
3. Explain the procedure to the patient.
4. Wash your hands.
5. Sit the patient up on the bed with their back supported and their neck flexed a little (Figure 23.3). If they cannot sit up, position them upright on one side.
6. Agree a signal that the patient can use to tell you to stop the procedure (e.g. a raised hand).
7. Put on gloves.
8. Estimate the length of NGT which you will need: hold the NGT from the tip of the nose to the earlobe and then the xiphisternum (bottom of breastbone, Figure 23.4). Choose the closest marker to this on the NGT.
9. Check that the nostrils look symmetrical and there are no polyps.
10. If it comes with one, check the guidewire is in the plastic tube.
11. Moisten the NGT with the lubricant and slowly advance it through one nostril.
12. If you meet resistance, withdraw and use the other nostril.
13. Keep checking that the patient is OK.
14. Ask the patient to gesture when the NGT is at the back of their throat.
15. Give the patient the water and ask them to swallow a mouthful. As they do this, advance the NGT to the predetermined point.
16. Aspirate from the tube with a syringe. Test the aspirate with litmus, it should be pH 1–5.5.
17. If the pH indicates that the NGT is in the correct place, tape it to the patient's face and secure a bile bag if it is to be used to drain the stomach contents.
18. Remove the guidewire if present.

Post-procedure

1. Document the procedure, the pH of the aspirate in the notes.
2. Arrange a chest X-ray to check the tube is in the stomach (Figure 23.5).
3. Inform nursing team that you have completed the procedure.

Contraindications to NGT insertion

- Head injury. If there is suspicion of a basal skull fracture, the NGT could theoretically enter the brain.
- Oesophageal stricture or obstruction
- Oesophageal varices
- Perforation of the gastrointestinal tract
- Clotting abnormality

Pitfalls

- Aspirate contains air but no fluid. This is probably because the NGT is not quite far enough in. Gently advance it and reaspirate.
- No air or aspirate. This may be because the NGT is against the stomach wall. Withdraw it a little and try again.
- Tube in lungs. This should not occur if the procedure is followed correctly. However, if the NGT has been inserted into the lungs, repositioning (as above) will not result in fluid being aspirated and the tube should be removed.

Top tips

- Pre-cool a Ryles tube in the refrigerator if possible. This makes it stiffer and more likely to pass in the correct direction. Make use of the tube's 'memory' to aid passage.
- Encourage the patient to keep the neck flexed (chin on chest) to again help the tube pass into the oesophagus and not the airway.

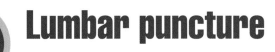

Lumbar puncture

24

Jane Sturgess

Figure 24.1 Equipment.

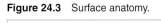

Figure 24.2 Patient position.

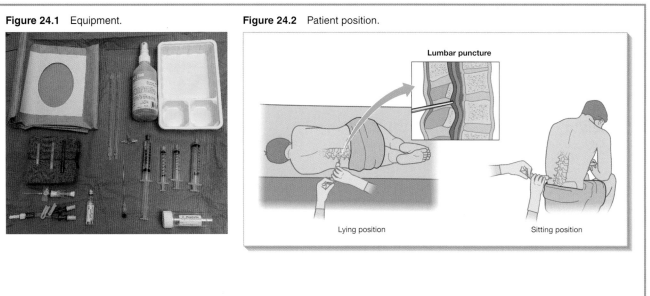

Lumbar puncture

Lying position

Sitting position

Figure 24.3 Surface anatomy.

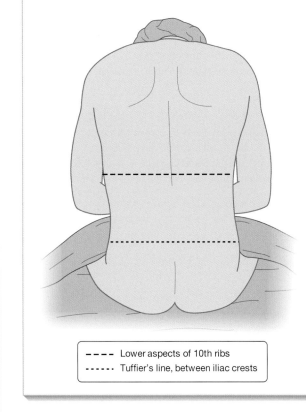

- – – – Lower aspects of 10th ribs
- ······· Tuffier's line, between iliac crests

Figure 24.4 Three-way tap and manometer.

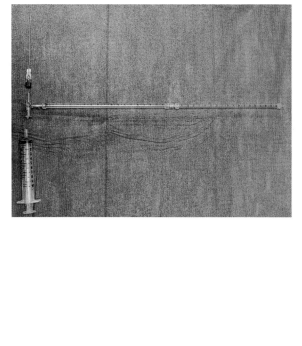

Applied Anatomy for Clinical Procedures at a Glance, First Edition. Jane Sturgess, Francesca Crawley, Ramez Kirollos, and Kirsty Cattle.
© 2021 John Wiley & Sons Ltd. Published 2021 by John Wiley & Sons Ltd.

Figure 24.5 Anatomical structures the needle will pass.

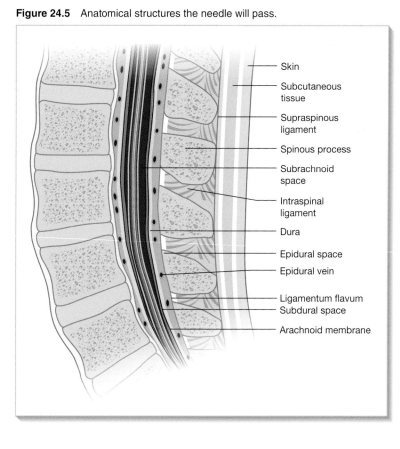

Skin

Subcutaneous tissue

Supraspinous ligament

Spinous process

Subrachnoid space

Intraspinal ligament

Dura

Epidural space

Epidural vein

Ligamentum flavum

Subdural space

Arachnoid membrane

Figure 24.6 Problems (a) bone only – articulated lumbar vertebrae, lordosis (b) bloody tap.

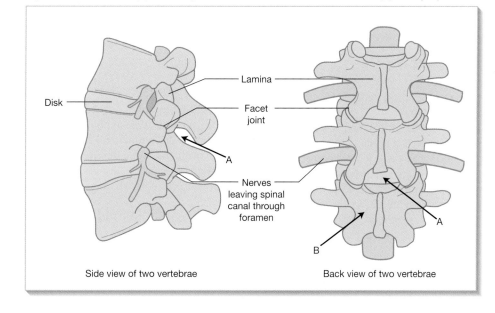

Disk

Lamina

Facet joint

A

Nerves leaving spinal canal through foramen

A

B

Side view of two vertebrae

Back view of two vertebrae

Equipment (Figure 24.1)

- Sterile field (Chapter 2), local anaesthetic (Chapter 5)
- Spinal needle 20 or 22 gauge, 3.8–8.9 cm length
- Manometer and three-way tap (see Chapters 3 and 7)
- 4 x sterile containers for samples (numbered 1–4) and sterile dressing
- Blood bottles for glucose, protein, and oligoclonal bands

Technique

1. Establish IV access and monitor oxygen saturation (SaO_2), electrocardiogram (ECG), and blood pressure (BP).
2. **Position** the patient in the left lateral position with their back parallel to the edge of the bed, the knees and hips flexed as far as possible, and the head and neck flexed (see Figure 24.2), or alternatively have the patient sitting, with their feet supported on a stool to flex the patient at their hips and knees, ask them to hug a pillow and put their chin onto their chest. These positions decrease the lumbar lordosis and open the interspinous space.
3. **Identify the L4/5 interspinous space** (see Figure 24.3).
4. Feel for the highest point of both iliac crests.
5. Draw (or imagine) a line between these points. This is called Tuffier's line and marks either the spinous process of L4 or the L4/5 interspinous space.
6. The lower aspects of the 10th rib correspond to the L1/2 interspace – a useful landmark in the obese patient.
7. It can be useful to mark the spaces above and below your intended needle insertion point.
8. **Prepare a sterile field**, scrub and prepare your surgical field (warn the patient that the skin preparation is cold, and the local anaesthetic stings).
9. Using a 25 gauge needle raise a skin wheal with up to 1 mL 1% lidocaine.
10. Insert a 20 gauge needle through the centre of the wheal to the hilt and use 5–10 mL 1% lidocaine to anaesthetise the deeper tissues as the needle is withdrawn towards the skin, aspirating before injecting.
11. Repeat this process in a couple of slightly different directions to ensure all tissue is numb.
12. This will allow you to get a 'feel' for the direction and depth you should aim for with the spinal needle.
13. Whilst waiting for the local anaesthetic to work **prepare your equipment** so that it is easy to get exactly what you want.
14. Connect the manometer to a three-way tap, and turn the tap to allow flow from the spinal needle to the manometer (Figure 24.4). It should be closed to air. This will allow you to attach it to the spinal needle as soon as cerebrospinal fluid (CSF) starts to flow.
15. Open your four sterile sample containers and label them with numbers 1–4.
16. **Insertion of the needle**. Remember the direction of the spinous processes and aim slightly cephalad.
17. Advance slowly and steadily. The needle passes through skin, subcutaneous fat, supraspinous ligament, interspinous ligament, ligamentum flavum, and finally dura (Figure 24.5). Your needle will be firmly gripped by the tissues when it sits in the interspinous ligament. You should feel a characteristic 'pop' as the dura is breached and CSF should flow. This is commonly at 4–5 cm.
18. Connect your manometer line and measure CSF opening pressure. Ensure the column of fluid is vertical to gain an accurate reading. Once CSF stops flowing up the manome-

ter read the level from the top of the meniscus (Figure 7.2). This is the pressure in cm of water.
19. Collect 10 drops of CSF into each numbered pot in order 1–4. Collect CSF for cell count, biochemistry (glucose, protein, and oligoclonal bands). Collect the oligoclonal bands in the last pot so it is least contaminated with blood.
20. Remove the needle (and introducer needle) in a single movement and apply gently pressure to the needle puncture site (especially if it is bleeding).
21. A small plaster or sterile spray can suffice as a dressing.
22. Place the patient supine and continue to monitor SaO_2, ECG, and BP. The patient can become hypotensive in response to the chemical sympathectomy induced by anaesthetising the lumbosacral sympathetic outflow if local anaesthetic is used.
23. Take blood for glucose, protein, and oligoclonal bands and send as paired samples with the CSF – timed and dated.

Aftercare

Bed rest after the procedure – to reduce CSF pressure, and possible CSF leak, leading to dural tap (or low pressure) headache

Common anatomical pitfalls

Bone only

- Off midline and hitting lamina only (Figure 24.6). Check insertion point and direction of needle tip to ensure in midline.
- Needle insertion angle too steep/too flat (see Figure 24.5).
- Poor positioning with inadequate flexion (see Figure 24.2), check patient well 'curled' with back straight along the edge of the bed.

Bloody tap

- Off midline and hitting epidural vessels (see Figure 24.5 and 24.6). If manometer clotted or no free flow of CSF try gentle flush of needle with 0.5 mL saline. If no improvement reposition needle.

CSF flow stops

- Needle tip has moved out of dural sac (see Figure 24.5). Check depth of needle, type of needle used (see Figure 24.1 showing location of the luminal exit) and either slowly advance or withdraw with the stylet removed from the needle. Sometimes rotating the needle 90 degrees can start flow again.
- Low CSF pressure. Ask the patient to perform a valsalva.

Obesity – unable to identify midline or spinous process

- Consider asking for anaesthetic or radiology opinion, or use of ultrasound or fluoroscopy.
- Consider using long needles.

Top tips

Position

- Make sure patient has their back perpendicular to the bed, and a good degree of flexion to open up the interspinous space and obliterate the lumbar lordosis.
- Left lateral (left side down, right side up) for right-handed operators. Right lateral for left handers allows easier manipulation of the needle.
- Sitting position can be useful if LP technically difficult – opening pressure inaccurate.

Insertion angle

- Remember the angle of the spinous processes – aiming for the umbilicus often helps.

Depth of dura

- In fit healthy patients it is unusual for you to need to insert the needle more than 6 cm. If you have not got CSF and are at the hilt of the needle you are likely to be off midline.

Preparation

- Having everything ready means you do not have to rotate to get equipment or take your eyes or hands off your needle. You are less likely to lose your direction.

- Keep bevel facing lateral to ease needle passage and cause less tissue damage (divides rather than cuts muscle fibres).

Position

- Normal CSF opening pressure measured in the lumbar region is dependent upon patient position. In the lateral position the pressure is commonly 10–18 cmH_2O, whereas it may be as great as 20–30 cmH_2O in the sitting position. Document the patient's position when measuring CSF opening pressure, so that repeat measurements can be made in the same position and results interpreted accordingly.

25 Bone marrow aspirate

Francesca Crawley and Charles Crawley

Figure 25.1 (a) Equipment trolley, including syringes, needles, cleaning pad, dressing, needle guards (red), BM aspirate needle with sternal guard in situ, BM trephine needle and trephine retrieval tools (yellow and green). (b) Frosted microscopy slides with bone marrow aspirate smears. Put the rest of the sample in an EDTA tube.

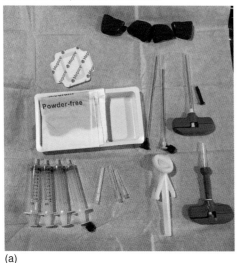

(a)

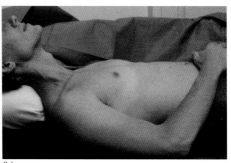

(b)

Figure 25.2 Patient position for (a) iliac crest or (b) sternal aspirate.

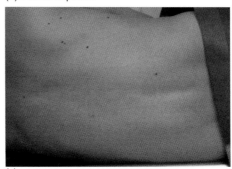

(a)

(b)

Figure 25.3 Posterior aspect of bony pelvis.

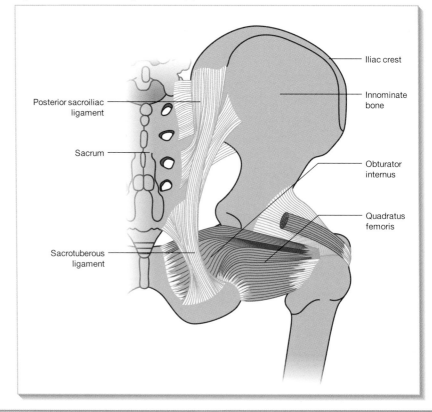

Posterior sacroiliac ligament

Sacrum

Sacrotuberous ligament

Iliac crest

Innominate bone

Obturator internus

Quadratus femoris

Applied Anatomy for Clinical Procedures at a Glance, First Edition. Jane Sturgess, Francesca Crawley, Ramez Kirollos, and Kirsty Cattle.
© 2021 John Wiley & Sons Ltd. Published 2021 by John Wiley & Sons Ltd.

Equipment (Figure 25.1)

- Alcohol-based skin antiseptic/iodine
- Dressing pack
- 2x sterile gloves
- 5x 10 or 20 mL syringes (practitioners preference)
- 2 x green needles
- 1x orange/blue needle (practitioners preference)
- 10 mL 2% lignocaine (lidocaine)
- Dressing towel
- Disposable marrow aspirate needle kit
- 5x frosted microscopy slides
- Pencil
- Slide holder and cover
- 3x full blood count (EDTA) tubes
- Cytogenetics pot (kept in refrigerator at -4 degrees
- Appropriate sample bottles if tuberculosis (TB) cultures requested
- Disposable trephine needle kit
- Container with formalin
- Plaster

Pre-procedure

Never perform a bone marrow aspirate without a trained member of staff (generally a nurse) to assist.

Identify patient and assemble equipment.

1. Check it is the correct patient by asking them to state their name. Obtain verbal consent. Check whether they are on any blood thinning medication (generally warfarin or aspirin). If they are, see notes opposite.
2. Ensure the patient is not allergic to lignocaine (lidocaine).
3. Obtain history from patient to avoid previous sites of radiotherapy.

Procedure

1. Assist the patient into the required position: on side or prone for iliac crest (see Figure 25.3 for anatomy), semirecumbent for sternal aspirate (Figure 25.2).
2. Clean site with alcohol-based skin antiseptic as per hospital policy.
3. Draw up 10 mL of lignocaine (lidocaine) into a 10 mL syringe with a green needle.
4. Change needle to orange/blue and inject 0.5 mL of local anaesthetic into the subcutaneous tissue, raising a blip over the intended site.
5. Wait 20 seconds for the anaesthetic to work.
6. Change the orange/blue needle to a green needle and penetrate tissue further until periosteum reached. Draw back to ensure not in a vein. Vary the direction of the needle and infiltrate the periosteum with local anaesthetic.
7. Wait 2–5 minutes for the local anaesthetic to work.
8. Before inserting the aspirate needle, ensure workstation is prepared to allow the first sample to be both spread for slide morphology and put into EDTA for flow cytometry. Aspirating repeated volumes of aspirate from the same place reduces the quality of morphology and flow cytometry analysis.
9. When the needle is in the bone marrow space a slight 'give' will be felt. Remove the introducer. Attach the 20 mL syringe, warn the patient that it will be uncomfortable but only for a few seconds, then suck quickly and aspirate not more than 0.5 mL of bone marrow and spread the marrow immediately onto the glass slides for **morphology** (make 5 slides). Put the rest of the content of the first aspirate syringe in an EDTA tube for morphology and flow cytometry. If a second aspirate is required, turn the needle 180 degrees and attach a second 30 mL syringe and aspirate a further 1–2 mL of bone marrow with appropriate warning to the patient. Put the content into the second EDTA tube for FISH (fluorescence in situ hybridisation) and **molecular** studies and the last 2 mL of bone marrow into the **cytogenetic** pot for karyotype studies (if required).
10. If TB cultures are requested, attach a 10 mL syringe and aspirate 10 mL of bone marrow. Put 5 mL of bone marrow in a special TB culture medium (bottle available from microbiology) and a further 5 mL into a plain universal tube.
11. Withdraw the needle; apply pressure and, assuming any bleeding has stopped, a plaster.
12. Take a blood sample in an EDTA tube to enable a blood film to be made.
13. Ensure specimens are correctly labelled and arrange safe and immediate transfer to haematology.

Clotting requirements for a bone marrow aspirate

1. Assess the platelet count and bleeding tendency of the patient. Patients with a history of bleeding, a diagnosis of myelodyplasia or receiving anti-platelets may require more detailed assessment prior to aspiration.
2. It is safe to do an aspirate, but not a trephine, with any platelet count.
3. If the patient is receiving low-molecular-weight heparin prophylactically, it is safe to perform an aspirate or trephine.
4. If the patient is receiving therapeutic anticoagulation it is safe to perform an aspirate or trephine as long as the International Normalised Ratio (INR) is <3 for warfarin and the activated partial thromboplastin time (APTT) ratio <2.5 on unfractionated heparin.

26 Ascitic tap

Francesca Crawley

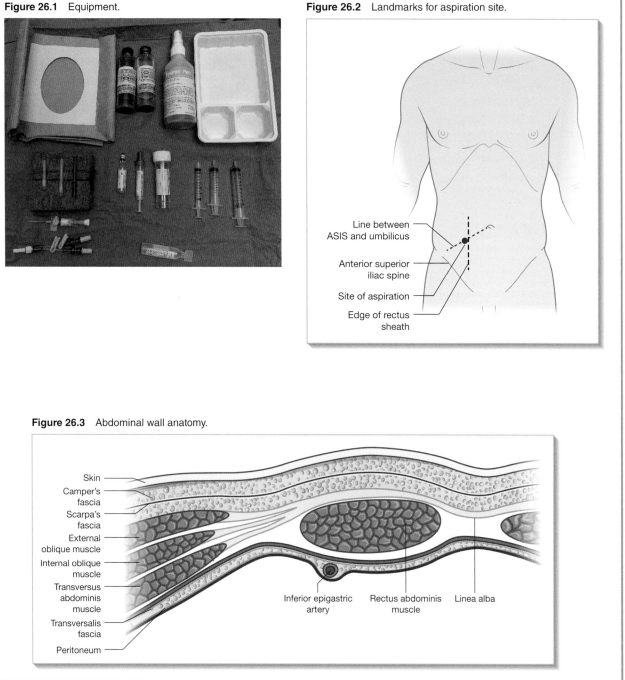

Figure 26.1 Equipment.

Figure 26.2 Landmarks for aspiration site.

Line between ASIS and umbilicus

Anterior superior iliac spine

Site of aspiration

Edge of rectus sheath

Figure 26.3 Abdominal wall anatomy.

Skin

Camper's fascia

Scarpa's fascia

External oblique muscle

Internal oblique muscle

Transversus abdominis muscle

Transversalis fascia

Peritoneum

Inferior epigastric artery

Rectus abdominis muscle

Linea alba

Applied Anatomy for Clinical Procedures at a Glance, First Edition. Jane Sturgess, Francesca Crawley, Ramez Kirollos, and Kirsty Cattle.
© 2021 John Wiley & Sons Ltd. Published 2021 by John Wiley & Sons Ltd.

Equipment (Figure 26.1)
- Sterile field pack (gloves, pack, and chlorhexidine swabs)
- Lignocaine 1% or 2%, 10 mL
- Green (19 gauge) and orange (25 gauge) needles
- 20 mL syringe with green (19 gauge) needle
- Sharps bin
- Universal specimen containers (×3) and EDTA blood bottle
- Blood culture bottles
- Dressing
- Ultrasound (if available)

Contraindications
- Abnormal clotting. Aim for the International Normalised Ratio (INR) to be 1.5 or less.
- Skin infection at tap site

Pre-procedure
1. Check patient's details, explain the procedure, and obtain consent.
2. Lay patient flat with their head on a pillow. Palpate/percuss for ascites. Confirm with ultrasound if available.
3. Palpate anterior superior iliac spine and visualise a point a third to halfway between this and the umbilicus. This can be on either side and must be lateral to rectus sheath (Figure 26.2).

Procedure
1. Check that you have established (by percussion, or if possible, use ultrasound) your site.
2. Clean skin with chlorhexidine swab and apply sterile drape.
3. Allow skin prep to dry and then use orange (25 gauge) needle to anaesthetise the skin.
4. Change to the green needle (19 gauge) and infiltrate deeper with lignocaine. Ensure that you withdraw before you inject (to avoid infiltrating a vessel). Do not use more than 10 mL of lignocaine.
5. Allow a few minutes for the lignocaine to work and then assemble a 20 mL syringe with a clean green (19 gauge) needle.
6. Advance the needle, aspirating after you have passed through skin. Continue to advance/aspirate until fluid is obtained. Withdraw 20 mL.
7. The needle passes through the skin, superficial fascia of Camper, the membranous layer of the superficial fascia of Scarpa, the external oblique muscle, the interior oblique muscle, the transversus abdominis, and then the peritoneum (Figure 26.3).
8. Apply sterile dressing and explain to the patient that the procedure is finished.

Post-procedure
1. Divide aspirate between EDTA bottle, blood culture bottles, and three universal containers (microbiology, biochemistry, and cytology – the largest should go to cytology). Label these.
2. Complete request forms.
3. Microbiology: microscopy, sensitivity, and culture. Mention if there is a possibility of tuberculosis (as this requires different processing).
4. Microbiology: inoculate both blood culture bottles with ascitic fluid.
5. Biochemistry: protein, albumin, lactate dehydrogenase (LDH), glucose (can also request amylase if appropriate).
6. Take blood for serum glucose, albumin, and LDH.

Top tips
- If you cannot clinically determine ascites (by percussion and/or palpation) use ultrasound or ask for senior help.
- In a large person a spinal needle can be used to infiltrate the lignocaine.
- If you hit a blood vessel when infiltrating with lignocaine, withdraw the needle and alter the skin position by about a centimetre and start again.
- You can use a larger (50 mL) syringe if you need a larger specimen (e.g. malignancy expected).
- If you have extra fluid, put it in a universal container and send to the biochemistry lab in case it is needed at a later date.

27 Paracentesis

Francesca Crawley

Figure 27.1 Equipment.

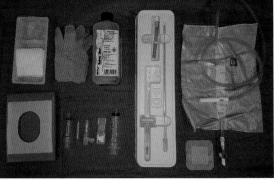

Figure 27.2 Landmarks for aspiration site.

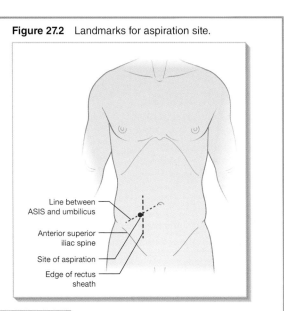

Line between ASIS and umbilicus

Anterior superior iliac spine

Site of aspiration

Edge of rectus sheath

Figure 27.3 Abdominal wall anatomy.

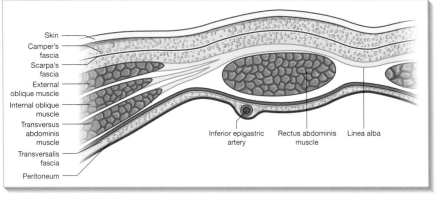

Skin

Camper's fascia

Scarpa's fascia

External oblique muscle

Internal oblique muscle

Transversus abdominis muscle

Transversalis fascia

Peritoneum

Inferior epigastric artery

Rectus abdominis muscle

Linea alba

Figure 27.4 'z' track to avoid overlapping skin and peritoneal puncture sites.

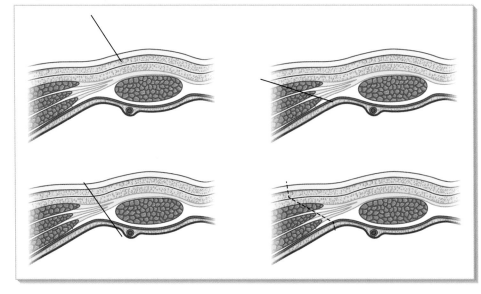

Applied Anatomy for Clinical Procedures at a Glance, First Edition. Jane Sturgess, Francesca Crawley, Ramez Kirollos, and Kirsty Cattle.
© 2021 John Wiley & Sons Ltd. Published 2021 by John Wiley & Sons Ltd.

Indications

- Patient with ascites with fever, encephalopathy, hypotension, or abdominal pain
- Symptomatic treatment of large volume ascites

Equipment (Figure 27.1)

- Sterile field pack (gloves, pack, and chlorhexidine swabs)
- Lignocaine 1% or 2%, 10 mL
- Green (19 gauge) and orange (25 gauge) needles
- 20 mL syringe with green (19 gauge) needle
- Sharps bin
- Dressing
- Ultrasound (if available)
- Paracentesis needle with multiple side perforations (or will get blocked by abdominal wall)
- Drainage tube
- Sealed sterile bottle to collect fluid

Pre-procedure

1. Check clotting. Aim for International Normalised Ratio (INR) of 1.5 or less.
2. Check patient's details, explain the procedure, and obtain consent.
3. Lay patient flat with their head on a pillow. Palpate/percuss for ascites. Confirm with ultrasound if available.

Procedure

1. The paracentesis site is generally the right lower quadrant of the abdominal wall (Figure 27.2).
2. Clean skin with chlorhexidine swab and apply sterile drape.
3. Allow skin prep to dry and then use orange (25 gauge) needle to anaesthetise the skin.
4. Change to the green needle (19 gauge) and infiltrate deeper with lignocaine. Ensure that you withdraw before you inject (to avoid infiltrating a vessel). Do not use more than 10 mL of lignocaine.
5. Allow a few minutes for the lignocaine to work and then assemble a 20 mL syringe with a clean green (19 gauge) needle.
6. Advance the needle, aspirating after you have passed through skin. Continue to advance/aspirate until fluid is obtained.

7. Then insert paracentesis needle perpendicular to the skin and advance through the subcutaneous fat and abdominal layers (see Figure 27.3) with the needle at about 45 degrees to skin. Ensure the needle is again perpendicular when the peritoneum is punctured. (This is a 'Z' track and ensures that the skin puncture and peritoneal sites do not overlap, see Figure 27.4.)
8. Aspirate as advancing the needle and stop when fluid is reached.
9. Thread the plastic tubing through the cannula until fluid runs through its lumen.
10. Withdraw the needle and attach the tubing to the bottle.
11. If fluid has ceased to flow advance the tubing a little until it does. Be sure to maintain sterile conditions.

Post-procedure

1. Fluid should be allowed to drain over 1–4 hours and the tubing should not be left overnight.
2. If drainage stops the patient should lie on the side of the drain to encourage further fluid to drain.
3. Once it is determined (by percussion/ultrasound) that the ascites has drained, remove the tubing and position the patient on their opposite side for two hours. If there is still leakage secure the site with a purse string suture.
4. Check your local guidelines, but if less than 5 litres has been withdrawn it is usual to replace this with a synthetic plasma expander such as gelofusine. If a larger volume has been removed, a volume expander (albumin) should be used in addition to the plasma expander. This is generally 8 g albumin per litre of ascites removed.

Complications

- Leak from puncture site
- Abdominal wall haematoma
- Bowel perforation
- Infection
- Hypotension after a large volume paracentesis
- Dilutional hypotension
- Hepatorenal syndrome
- Major blood vessel laceration

28 Knee aspiration

Sherif Kirollos and Ramez Kirollos

Figure 28.1 Equipment.

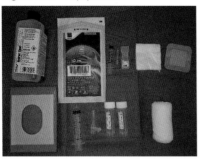

Figure 28.2 Knee surface anatomy with approaches for knee arthrocentesis.

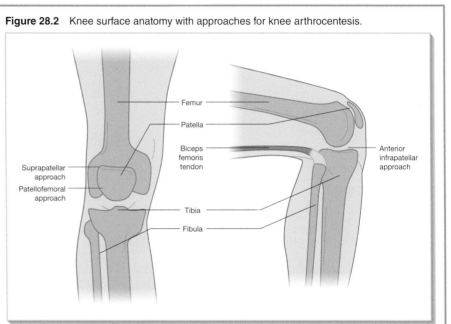

Figure 28.3 Lateral anatomy of knee.

Figure 28.4 Bursae around the knee joint.

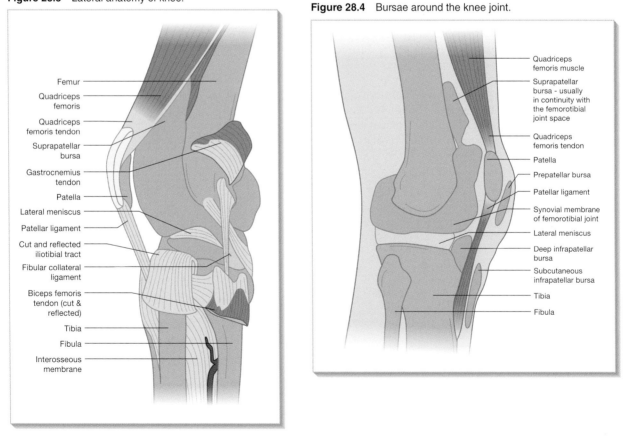

Applied Anatomy for Clinical Procedures at a Glance, First Edition. Jane Sturgess, Francesca Crawley, Ramez Kirollos, and Kirsty Cattle.
© 2021 John Wiley & Sons Ltd. Published 2021 by John Wiley & Sons Ltd.

Equipment (Figure 28.1)

- Sterile gloves
- Antiseptic solution for skin preparation
- Fenestrated sterile towel
- Local anaesthetic, needle, and syringe
- Needle, 18 to 21 gauge, approximately 4 cm in length
- Gauze
- Sterile containers for collection of samples
- Sterile dressing
- Elastic bandage

Indications

- Diagnostic
  - Suspicion of septic arthritis
  - Unexplained knee effusion
  - Arthropathies such as differentiating gout from pseudogout
- Therapeutic
  - Provide relief from large painful effusions
  - Injections of steroids or antibiotics

Procedure

1. Check your equipment.
2. Prepare the skin with antiseptic solution and drape.
3. Administer local anaesthetic.
4. For a femorotibial joint approach, place the knee in slight flexion (15–20 degrees) to open up the joint space by placing a folded towel underneath. This also keeps the quadriceps muscle relaxed.
5. A prominent supra- or parapatellar swelling will determine the entry point.
6. There are several approaches to knee arthrocentesis (Figure 28.2):
   a. Patellofemoral approaches
      - Through a medial or lateral entry point adjacent to the middle border of the patella with the knee in extension and the patella pulled in the direction away from the entry point. The needle is directed 45 degrees towards the midline deep to the patella to access the patellofemoral joint.
   b. Suprapatellar approaches
      - Used in the presence of a large effusion of the suprapatellar bursa with the entry point at the superomedial or superolateral corner of the patella. The needle is then directed deep to the patellar articular surface with the knee in extension.
   c. Anterior infrapatellar approaches
      - The knee is flexed and the entry point is either lateral or medial to the patellar tendon (between patella and tibial tuberosity) and thus avoiding the extensor mechanism. The needle is then directed into the femorotibial joint between the femoral condyle and tibial plateau with care to avoid damage to the menisci and articular cartilage. This is similar to the approach for knee arthroscopy and used in cases of minimal effusion.
7. Following aspiration, send the aspirate to the appropriate laboratories for analysis.

Aftercare

- If haemarthrosis occurs this is usually minor and self-limiting.

Common anatomical pitfalls (Figure 28.3)

- The needle's tip is placed in the patellofemoral joint (where a non-communicating bursa is punctured) rather than the femorotibial joint.
- The suprapatellar bursa may not communicate with the knee joint.
- Avoid penetrating the patellar tendon if aspirating inferior to the patella by keeping at the lateral inferior angles of the patella.
- Stop deep advancement of the needle once the fluid is aspirated to avoid damage of the articular cartilage.
- Avoid aspiration in the presence of overlying cellulitis.

Anatomical top tips

- Normally the suprapatellar bursa is an extension of the synovial capsule and extends 2 finger breadths above the top of the patella.
- Aspirating a prosthetic joint, should ideally be discussed with the orthopaedic team as introduction of infection will have disastrous consequences.
- Ultrasound-guidance may improve the accuracy of aspirations and injections.
- Note that several bursae surrounding the knee joint do not communicate with the joint space (Figure 28.4). This includes the superficial and deep infrapatellar bursa and the prepatellar bursa.

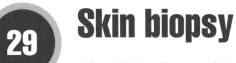

Skin biopsy

Sherif Kirollos and Ramez Kirollos

Figure 29.1   Equipment.

Figure 29.2   Skin layers.

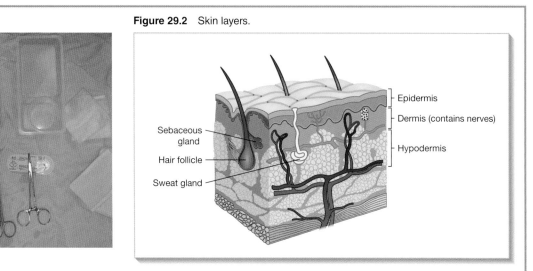

- Epidermis
- Dermis (contains nerves)
- Hypodermis

Sebaceous gland
Hair follicle
Sweat gland

Figure 29.3   Shave biopsy. Holding the blade almost horizontal to the skin "shave" the lesion for biopsy off the healthy underlying skin.

Figure 29.4   Punch biopsy. (a) The punch. (b) In use.

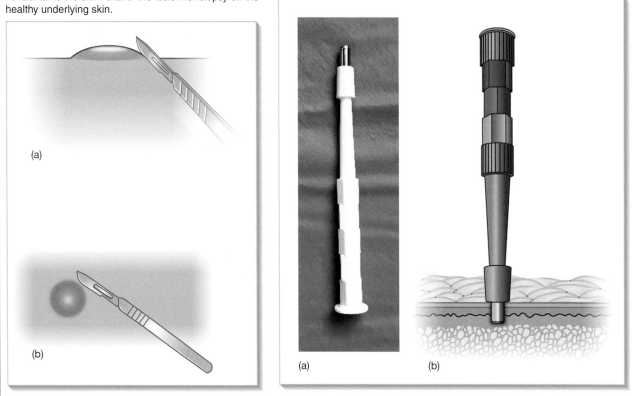

(a)

(b)

(a)

(b)

Applied Anatomy for Clinical Procedures at a Glance, First Edition. Jane Sturgess, Francesca Crawley, Ramez Kirollos, and Kirsty Cattle.
© 2021 John Wiley & Sons Ltd. Published 2021 by John Wiley & Sons Ltd.

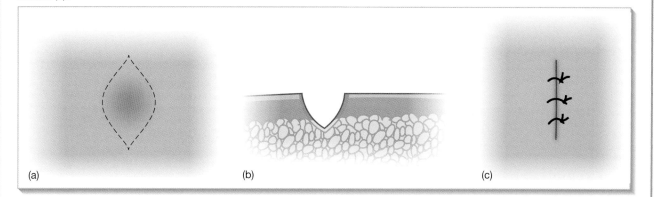

Figure 29.5 Excision biopsy. (a) Make an elliptical incision around the lesion, down to the subcutaneous fat (b). Close the defect with sutures (c).

(a)   (b)   (c)

Equipment (Figure 29.1)
- Antiseptic solution
- Local anaesthetic
- Gloves
- Toothed forceps
- Sutures
- Scissors
- Needle holder
- Gauze
- Container for tissue samples
- Biopsy punch (for punch biopsies)
- Scalpel with number 15 blade (for shave and excisional biopsies)

Indications
- Diagnosis of pigmented skin lesions
- Diagnosis of suspected skin cancers
- Certain dermatological conditions

Procedure
1. Prepare the skin with alcohol wipes, povidone-iodine, or chlorhexidine and administer local anaesthetic. A fenestrated surgical drape should be placed over the biopsy site if performing an excisional biopsy.
2. There are various skin biopsy techniques depending on the indication for the biopsy and the configuration of the lesion (Figure 29.2):
   a. Shave biopsy (Figure 29.3)
      - Used for elevated skin lesions such as skin tags or warts, or those not extending deep to the epidermis such as superficial squamous or basal cell carcinomas.
      - After injecting local anaesthetic around the lesion, a 15 blade scalpel is used parallel to the skin surface at the base of the lesion and the lesion is superficially excised while avoiding angulating the blade to the deep tissues. Alternatively curved scissors may be used.
      - Haemostasis is usually achieved just by applying local pressure.
   b. Punch biopsy (Figure 29.4)
      - This is often indicated for the removal of small lesions or biopsy of the centre or edge of larger lesions.
      - Stretch the skin perpendicular to the skin tension lines around the lesion which may be outlined using a marker. This will allow the defect to undertake an elliptical form following the biopsy, permitting a superior cosmetic result following healing.
      - Position the punch biopsy tool (which has a round knife with varying diameters although 3 mm achieves the balance between obtaining histological diagnosis and an acceptable cosmetic result, Figure 29.4a) directly over the lesion and apply a downward pressure in a rotational motion until a 'give' is felt, indicating passage to the subcutaneous tissue. The base of the core is divided and the sample is retrieved. Apply pressure to achieve haemostasis.
   c. Excisional biopsy (Figure 29.5)
      - Use a field block by local anaesthesia.
      - Leaving a generous margin of approximately 2–5 mm around the lesion, create an elliptical incision around the lesion using a number 15 blade. Ensure the incision is deep enough to reach the subcutaneous fat.
      - Once the elliptical incision with its long axis parallel to the tension lines has been made, use forceps to lift up the lesion at its edges and undercut the sample with the scalpel.
      - Suture the wound in layers and apply a dressing.
      - Send the sample to the appropriate laboratory for analysis.

Anatomical pitfalls
- Avoid a punch biopsy in areas in proximity to superficial nerves such as the digital nerves.

Top tips
- If biopsying a cancerous lesion, avoid obtaining a punch biopsy.
- An excisional biopsy rather than other types of biopsies should be performed in cases of pigmented lesions suspicious of melanoma and should include the deep layers (subcutaneous fat) to allow staging of the lesion. Deeper histological extension of a melanoma may require wider re-excision of the margins.
- When presented with multiple lesions, in most circumstances it is best to biopsy those which demonstrate the most advanced inflammatory changes as biopsying a lesion at a very early stage is likely to show nonspecific features. Conversely, it presented with a blistering lesion, histology reveals greater specificity in lesions at an early stage of development.
- Either biopsy the centre or excise the entire lesion for lesions smaller than 4 mm in diameter. For large lesions, biopsy the edge, the thickest portion, or the area that is most abnormal in color, to increase the diagnostic yield as these sites will most likely contain the distinctive pathological features.
- Smooth movements are performed during obtaining a punch biopsy as back-and-forth twisting motions or intermittently removing the punch to check the progress may result in a ragged wound edge and a macerated biopsy sample.

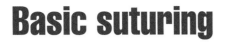

30 Basic suturing

Sherif Kirollos and Ramez Kirollos

Figure 30.1 Equipment. Needle holder, suture scissors, appropriate suture material.

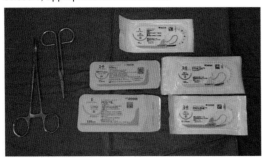

Figure 30.2 How to mount a needle. Note the needle is mounted at the junction of ⅓ and ⅔ along the needle.

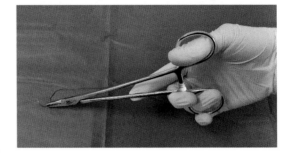

Figure 30.3 Different suturing techniques. (a) Inverted/buried sutures. (b) Transverse/vertical mattress sutures. (c) Running/continuous sutures. (d) Interlocking continuous sutures. (e) Figure of eight sutures, e.g. to join tendon ends or close a laparoscopy incision. (f) Stapler and stapling.

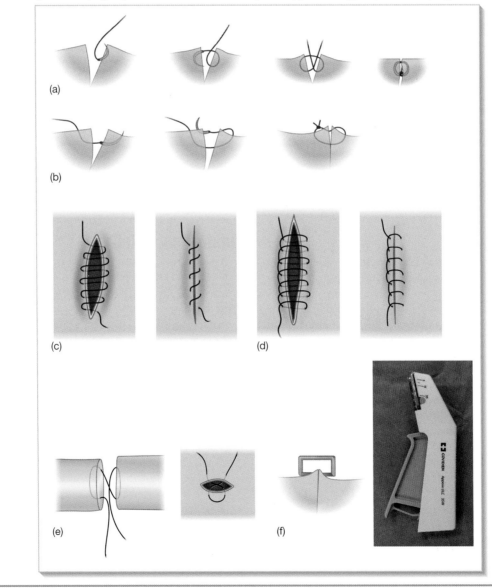

Applied Anatomy for Clinical Procedures at a Glance, First Edition. Jane Sturgess, Francesca Crawley, Ramez Kirollos, and Kirsty Cattle.
© 2021 John Wiley & Sons Ltd. Published 2021 by John Wiley & Sons Ltd.

Equipment (Figure 30.1)
- Suture
- Needle holder
- Suture scissors

Choice of suture
- Suture materials
  - Absorbable vs. non-absorbable
    Absorbable sutures are degraded gradually by tissue enzymes and this process is associated with varying degrees of tissue reaction and scar formation. Natural sutures material are associated with excessive tissue inflammatory reaction.
  - Braided vs. non-braided
    Braided sutures are strands of suture material twisted together. Braided sutures have the advantage of allowing easier and more secure knot tying but are more liable to harbour bacteria and may hence increase the risk of infection.
- Tensile strength
  Is the ability of the material to resist the maximum longitudinal stress to prevent it from breaking apart.

	Absorbable	Non-absorbable
Natural	Catgut (collagen)	Silk
Synthetic	Polyglactin 910 (Vicryl)	Nylon (Ethilon)
	Polyglycolic acid (Dexon)	Polypropylene (Prolene)
	Polydioxanone (PDS)	

- Types of needles
  The shape of the needle could be curved (with varying degrees of curvature) or straight. Straight needles are less likely used and generally do not require a needle holder during suturing.
    The tip of the needle can be cutting with a sharp tapered tip and sharp edges (facilitated penetration of tough tissues such as skin and fascia) or round bodied (atraumatic used for example in anastomosis, for mucous membranes, subcutaneous tissues).
- Size of suture and needles
  Suture sizes varies from 00 (thick) to 10/0 (hair like) and the bigger suture sizes are associated with bigger needles. Large sizes are stronger and used for example in abdominal closure while fine sutures are used for microsurgical procedures such as small vessel anastomosis and some ophthalmological procedures. A 4/0 or 5/0 sutures are recommended to be used on the face for cosmetic reasons.

Factors determining the choice of sutures and needles
- Handling. Monofilament sutures on atraumatic needles for delicate tissues and vascular anastomosis. The use of different needle sizes and varying curvatures is adapted to the configuration and depth of the tissue to be sutured.
- Strength. Large suture (on larger needles) offers more secure and stronger closure. Cutting needles pass easier through stronger fascial layers.
- Knot security. Braided > monofilament
- Potential of infection. Braided > monofilament

Technique
General principles
1. The needle is ideally held on the needle holder one third of the distance from its base to the tip up to midpoint (Figure 30.2). Avoid distorting the curvature of the needle during handling. The edge of the incision to be sutured is slightly everted by gently holding it with forceps in the other hand without crushing the edge. This allows that the entrance of the needle is perpendicular to the surface and include the full thickness. The needle is then passed similarly through the other edge from deep to surface either in a single maneuver or retrieving the needle first in the depth of the wound and then remounting it on the needle holder and pass again through the second edge. The surgeon's wrist movements should follow the curve of the needle. While pulling the needle out be sure not to hold its tip by the needle holder so as not to damage or render the tip blunt for subsequent use. Similarly avoid holding the base of the needle/suture junction as this may break.

2. The bites, whether using interrupted or continuous sutures, should be symmetrical on both sides and about 3–5 mm from the edge depending on the tissue to be sutured and spaced symmetrically 5–10 mm along the length. Ensure that the full thickness on either side is included and with perpendicular needle entrance and exit that no inversion or eversion of the edges occur. The edges should hence by perfectly opposed and this also necessitate that the tension applied on tying the knots is adequate enough for this purpose without being either loose or strangulating the tissue so that will not compromise the local blood supply.

3. The knot is tied using three throws in alternating different directions for most suture materials. However, for monofilament nylon or Prolene suture six throws may be required to avoid slippage of the knot.

4. Suturing of skin may include the epidermis and dermis in one layer and the subcutaneous fat as a separate deeper layer. Suturing of mucous membranes requires delicate tissue handling and avoid tight sutures that may potentially cut through the sutured membrane as these tissues are liable for excessive postoperative swelling. Fine absorbable sutures on atraumatic round bodied needles are used.

Variations in suturing techniques
1. Inverted/buried sutures (Figure 30.3a). These allow the knot to be buried from the surface. The needle is first passed from deep to superficial on one side and then from superficial to deep on the other side before the knot is tied. May be used for the muscle or subcutaneous fat layers.
2. Transverse mattress sutures (Figure 30.3b). These are beneficial whenever there is difficulty in preventing inversion of the edges so as to achieve apposition of the skin edges. This situation may be encountered during suturing a reopened incision that has developed scar tissue at its edges from the initial surgery. After passing the needle through both edges as in a simple suture the direction of the needle is reversed and passed nearer to the edge of the side where it exited from outside in and then from inside out near the edge of the contralateral side and the knot is tied on the initial side.
3. Running/continuous sutures (Figure 30.3c). Should ensure that the edges are opposed throughout the length of the sutured incision. These achieve haemostatic control of bleeding skin edges in hypervascular regions.
4. Interlocking continuous sutures (Figure 30.3d). A variation of continuous suturing wherein on one side the thread is interlocked through the previous throw before passing again through both edges. This achieves even more efficient haemostasis from the bleeding edges.
5. Figure-of-eight sutures (Figure 30.3e). Used to approximate tissues with a gap such as in the repair of torn tendons and occasionally other tissues such as muscles and skin.

6. Staples (Figure 30.3f). Placing metal staples using an applicator across the wound or incision approximates the edges in a quick fashion with advantages of rapid control of bleeding edges such as the scalp. Due to the possible resulting skin marks should be avoided on the face. Again the edges are slightly everted and approximated with forceps and the staples applied with applicator centered on the incision line to allow the staples to lie symmetrically on either edge. A 10 mm gap between staples is acceptable.

Removal of sutures

• Non-absorbable skin sutures should be removed in a timely fashion to minimise scarring. Skin sutures are removed after 7–10 days and those on the face in 3–5 days. A staple removal instrument is required to remove staples when used.

Anatomical pitfalls

• Recognising strong holding structures. In deep incisions it is the fascia that represents the strong layer that is responsible for the strength of the wound. Adequate placement of sutures in this layer depends upon identification of its edges which may be retracted within the incised layers.

• Loose suturing. The proper tension while tying the knots of the sutures results in apposition of the edges to allow healing and without compromise of the blood supply. Failure of applying adequate tension of failure to suture the structures giving strength to the closure such as the fascia and skin can have adverse consequences such as a burst abdomen.

• Strangulating suturing. The purpose is to approximate tissues or incised edges to allow healing. Excessive tension would potentially compromise the blood supply and hinders the healing process. Blanching of the skin edges while suturing indicates excessive tension. Muscle fibres should be only loosely approximated to allow for postoperative swelling.

• Blood supply compromise. In cases of vascularised flaps suturing the corners and even the distal edges by using full thickness sutures may compromise the blood supply as these are the most vulnerable parts of the flap being most distal from the vascular pedicle. This would compromise the healing resulting in wound dehiscence. A partial thickness suture such as an inverted subdermal suture approximating the edges and supplemented by steristrips applied to the skin would be advantageous.

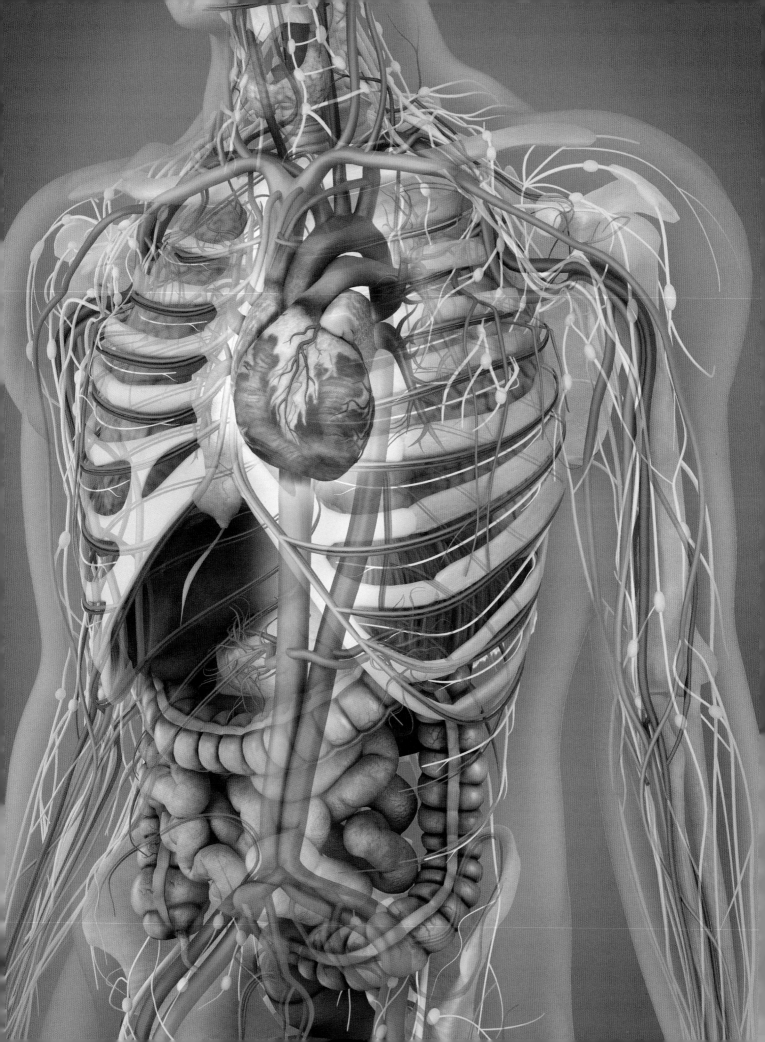

31 Basic anastomotic techniques

Sherif Kirollos and Ramez Kirollos

Figure 31.1a Equipment for bowel anastomosis.

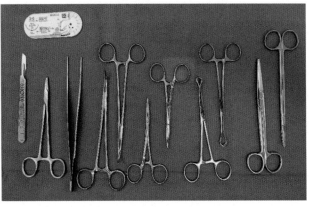

Figure 31.1b Equipment for vascular anastomosis.

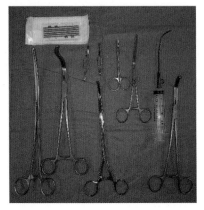

Figure 31.1c Stapling devices used for bowel anastomosis. © Ethicon, Inc. Reproduced with permission.

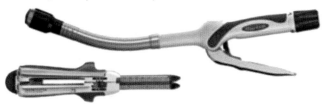

Figure 31.2 Different configurations of possible anastomoses, e.g. (a) end to end, (b) end to side, (c) side to side, (d) alternative side to side.

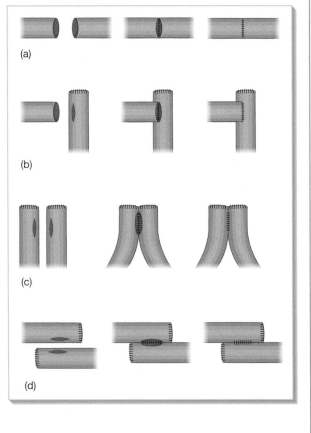

(a)

(b)

(c)

(d)

Figure 31.3 Posterior view of mesenteric vasculature.

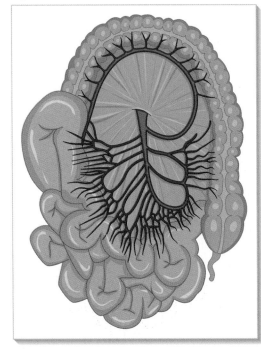

Applied Anatomy for Clinical Procedures at a Glance, First Edition. Jane Sturgess, Francesca Crawley, Ramez Kirollos, and Kirsty Cattle.
© 2021 John Wiley & Sons Ltd. Published 2021 by John Wiley & Sons Ltd.

Equipment (Figure 31.1a–c)

- Sutures
- Scalpel
- Needles
- Needle holders
- Forceps
- Scissors
- Bipolar coagulation
- Vascular clamps
- Vascular slings
- Irrigating syringes
- Stapling devices

Definition: connection of two tubular/hollow organs together, connecting one lumen to another lumen

Technique

- See Chapter 30 for principles of good suturing techniques.
- The edges are connected by either interrupted or continuous sutures. The advantage of interrupted sutures is the relative ease of placement with less manipulation of the edges due to better visualisation. However, this may require more time to accomplish as each suture is tied separately. The advantage for continuous sutures is speed in experienced hands.
- For bowel anastomosis sutures may be interrupted or continuous and the bites are either full thickness single or a double-layered closure. The edges should be well prepared, adequately mobilised to avoid tension on the anastomosis and well vascularised. Slowly absorbable monofilament sutures are preferred. Stapled anastomosis, especially in confined places such as the pelvis for colorectal anastomosis, are more commonly used.
- For vascular anastomosis, systemic anticoagulants are given during the procedure and the area is regularly irrigated and flushed using heparinised saline. The initial sutures at either end are placed from inside out using a double needle suture to prevent intimal 'flaps' and for the same reason ensure that all sutures are taken through the full thickness of the wall. Avoid constriction of the lumen or even suturing both walls together. Use fine monofilament sutures either interrupted or continuous. Bites should be symmetrical and avoid excessive gaps.

Types (Figure 31.2)

- End to end
- End to side
- Side to side

Anatomical pitfalls: Bowel

- Compromise of blood supply: The mesentery carries the blood supply (Figure 31.3). The arteries form anastomotic arches within the mesentery, which give rise to vasa recta which proceed to the border of the gut where they pass alternatively to supply opposite sides of the wall and end as fine arborisations forming an anti-mesenteric anastomosis. The sutures anastomosing both ends should not be tied with excessive tension so as not to strangulate the blood supply. Careful handling of the mesentery should be observed during mobilisation. Avoid excessive rotation that may cause kinking which may compromise the arterial supply or venous drainage.
- Leakage from an anastomosis
  - General causes
    - Presence of persistent distal obstruction
    - Poor healing from malnutrition or generalised sepsis
    - Underlying aetiology such as resection for ischaemic colitis or stricture repair in cases of radiation enteritis
  - Technical causes
    - Unrecognised loose sutures or gaps
    - Compromise of vascularity

Anatomical pitfalls: Vascular

- Intimal dissection
  - Attention to technical details to avoid creation of an intimal flap
- Leak
  - Each edge is neatly cut and prepared.
  - Remove tissues surrounding the adventitia.
  - Adequate mobilisation of both vessel ends to allow approximation without tension.
  - Attention to technical details. Avoid 'crushing' the edges by mishandling.
- Occlusion and thromboembolism
  - Damage on the intima due to mishandling
  - Intimal flaps
  - Inadequate or mistimed administration of anticoagulants/antiplatelets
  - Accidental suturing of the vessel's back wall

Aftercare: Bowel

- Diversion of contents
- Eliminate the possibility of distal obstruction

Aftercare: Vascular

- Anticoagulation/antiplatelets
- Monitor for distal ischaemia

32 Abscess drainage and debridement

Sherif Kirollos and Ramez Kirollos

Figure 32.1 Equipment.

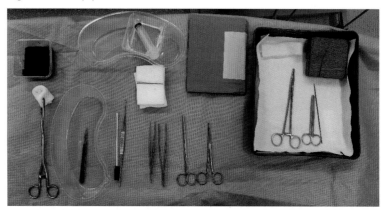

Figure 32.2 Procedure: (a) infiltrate region with local anaesthetic, (b) make incision over point of maximal fluctuance/where abscess is 'pointing', (c) take pus swab, (d) open all loculations with haemostat or finger, (e) irrigate with saline, (f) pack cavity and apply dressing.

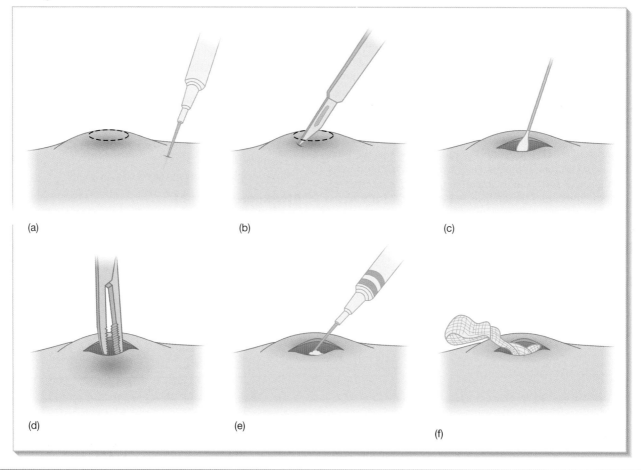

(a)

(b)

(c)

(d)

(e)

(f)

Applied Anatomy for Clinical Procedures at a Glance, First Edition. Jane Sturgess, Francesca Crawley, Ramez Kirollos, and Kirsty Cattle.
© 2021 John Wiley & Sons Ltd. Published 2021 by John Wiley & Sons Ltd.

Figure 32.3 Breast anatomy, showing lactiferous ducts.

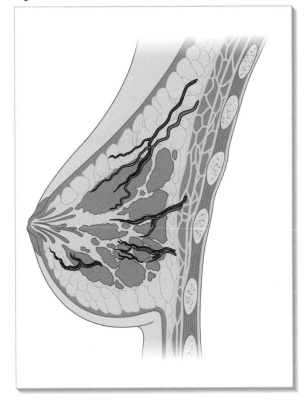

Figure 32.4 Park's classification of perianal abscesses: (1) Intersphincteric, (2) Transphincteric, (3) Suprasphincteric, (4) Extrasphincteric.

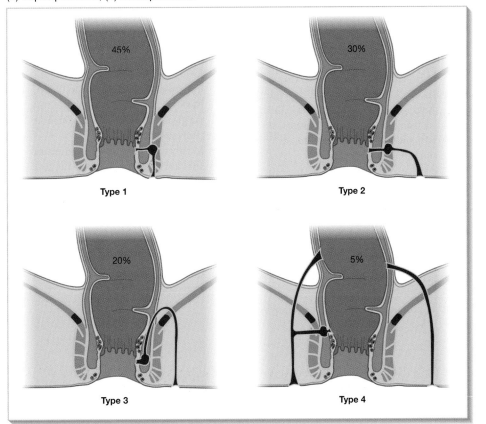

Equipment (Figure 32.1)

- Antiseptic solution
- Drapes
- Local anaesthetic
- Sterile gauze
- Syringe and needle
- Scalpel with size 11 blade
- Small curved haemostat
- Packing gauze
- Containers for microbiological samples
- Microbiological swabs

Procedure (Figure 32.2)

1. Anaesthetise the area of incision with local anaesthetic infiltration. The low pH in the abscess cavity may negate the analgesic effect of the local anaesthetic and hence additional sedation may be required.
2. Make an incision over the most prominent area of the abscess. Ensure the incision is deep enough to transgress the abscess wall and the opening is large enough to adequately drain the pus and to prevent recurrence of the abscess.
3. For cosmetic reasons, the long axis of the incision should be parallel to the skin tension line.
4. Loculations should be broken either via a haemostat or introduction of the fingertip to ensure drainage of pus from different pockets.
5. A microbiological swab sample and pus aspiration by syringe should be sent for microbiological analysis.
6. Following drainage, thoroughly irrigate the abscess cavity with normal saline.
7. Finally, consider packing the abscess with iodoform antiseptic impregnated ribbon gauze. This is to ensure the abscess is kept open to allow further drainage. Packing is performed only if needed and considered in large abscess cavities. Cover the abscess site with a non-adherent dressing.

Aftercare

- Antibiotics may be used especially in patients presenting with systemic features of sepsis. This would be altered depending on the culture and sensitivity results. In these cases, clinical and laboratory monitoring using inflammatory markers, such as C-reactive protein (CRP) and white cell count, dictates the period of antibiotic use and monitors progress.
- Regular inspection of the abscess site is imperative as a repeat incision and drainage may be required in some cases.
- When packing is used, this should be inspected and removed within 2–3 days. Occasionally in larger abscess cavities, repacking with a shorter length of ribbon gauze may be required for a further period of time. The abscess cavity is expected to heal by secondary intention.

Pitfalls

- In cases where there is an absence of pus drainage following the incision, consider:
  - The possibility of intervention during the cellulitis stage prior to abscess formation.
  - The incision has either not been made at the appropriate site or has been made too superficial in the case of a deep-seated abscess.
- Failure to drain loculated pus
- Failure to recognise and remove a foreign body in the abscess cavity
- Inadequate attention to precipitating factors such as control of blood-glucose in diabetic patients or underlying osteomyelitis

Anatomical top tips

- Drainage of breast abscess
  - The possible diagnostic pitfalls include the differential diagnosis of inflammatory carcinoma and mastitis stage before abscess formation.
  - The axis of the incision for drainage is best oriented radially from the areola at the site where the abscess is pointing to avoid disruption of multiple lactiferous ducts (Figure 32.3). There are 15–20 lactiferous ducts.
  - As the mammary gland is a modified subcutaneous gland there are fibrous septae attached between the deep skin and fascia (suspensory ligaments) and complete drainage of a large abscess requires opening the different pockets by using a haemostat through the incision.
  - Especially for deep lying abscess cavities, percutaneous needle aspiration under ultrasound guidance is advocated. An 18–22 gauge needle is used depending on the consistency of the pus. The procedure may be repeated as indicated. More recently, many recommend this over open incision and drainage.
  - The aftercare of 'lactating' abscess necessitates mechanical milk expression and suppression of lactation.
  - Subareolar infections (possible underlying mammary duct ectasia) may require a circumareolar incision for cosmetic reasons.
- Drainage of perianal abscess
  - Recognise underlying fistulae in cases of recurrent abscesses and possible relationship to Crohn's disease.
  - Most perianal abscesses are pointing subcutaneously and are surgically drained using the standard technique as described previously.
  - Mostly these arise from an infection of one of the anal glands that are located mainly at the level of the dentate line and extend to the internal anal sphincter (Figure 32.4).
  - Other regions of extension included are through the external anal sphincter to the ischiorectal fossa or less commonly to the intersphincteric groove between the internal sphincter which is in continuity of the inner circular muscle of the rectal wall and the external sphincter. However, extension to other spaces may be identified by preoperative investigations such as CT scans.

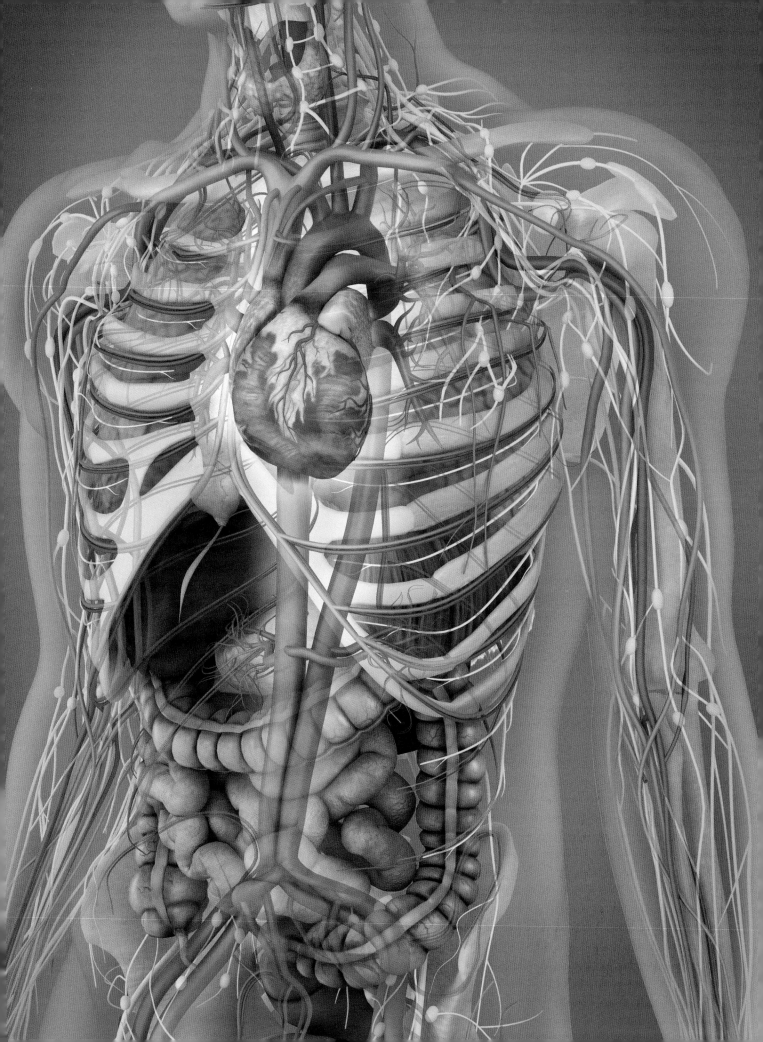

33 | Bag mask ventilation (adults)

Jane Sturgess

Figure 33.1 Equipment.

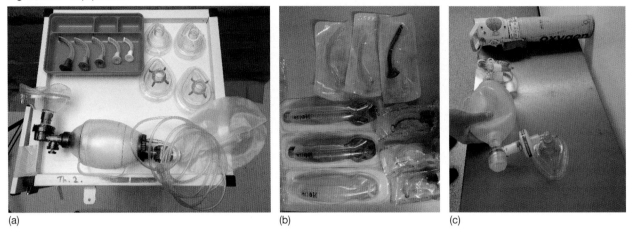

(a)　　　　　　　　　　　　　　(b)　　　　　　　　　　　　　　(c)

Figure 33.2 (a) Patient position – 'sniffing the morning air'. (b) Technique, showing operator finger placement and direction of force to gain a good seal and open the airway.

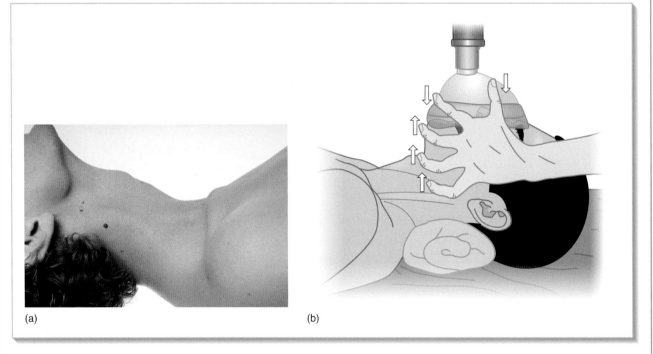

(a)　　　　　　　　　　　　　　　　　　(b)

Figure 33.3 Sagittal section of the open airway.

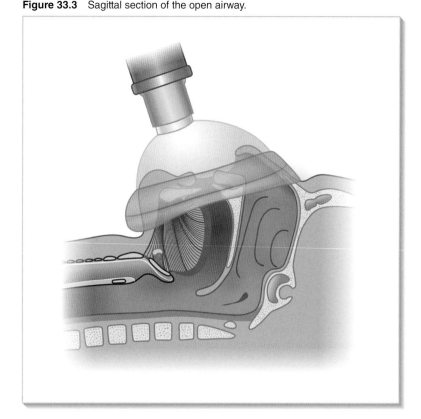

Equipment (Figure 33.1)

- Facemask size 3, 4, and 5
- Heat and moisture exchange (HME) filter
- Angle piece catheter mount
- Ambu Bag (1300 mL)
- Guedel airways size 2, 3, and 4
- Nasopharyngeal airways size 6, 7, 8, and 9
- Supraglottic airway size 3, 4, and 5
- A second person to squeeze the 'bag'

Technique (Figure 33.2)

1. Check your equipment.
2. Place the patient in the 'sniffing the morning air' position, neck flexed, head extended (Figure 33.2a).
3. Hold the facemask in both hands and place the apex of the triangle on the bridge of the nose. Keep in place with your thumbs.
4. Place your second and third fingers along the jaw line and pull the chin upwards towards the mask.
5. Use your index fingers to secure the lower part of the facemask tightly against the chin.
6. You should be pushing down towards the pillow with your thumbs and index fingers and pulling upwards (into the mask) with your remaining fingers (Figure 33.2b).
7. To further open the airway, place the tip of your little fingers behind the angle of the mandible and perform a jaw thrust.
8. If needed use an appropriately sized oropharyngeal or nasopharyngeal airway to ensure a patent airway.
9. Ask your assistant to squeeze the bag and deliver a breath.

Aftercare

- Bag mask ventilation (BMV) should be continued until return of spontaneous ventilation or until intubation.

- The ventilatory gases should be humidified and warmed for any ventilation longer than 30 minutes; placing an HME into the breathing circuit can achieve this.
- If a mask is to be fitted for a prolonged period of time, for example, CPAP in ventilatory failure or overnight in obstructive sleep apnoea, consider the need to take measures to preserve tissue integrity in pressure areas, specifically the nasal bridge.

Common anatomical pitfalls

- Placing the mask upside down will not achieve a good fit and makes maintaining a patent airway difficult; see Figure 33.3 for illustration of good position.
- Not placing the apex of the mask triangle at the bridge of the nose and squashing the nose occludes the airway.
- Choosing an ill-fitting mask will result in a large air leak and poor ventilation of the lungs.
- Poor head position will fail to align the trachea. High pressure or large tidal volume breaths are used to counteract this problem but the result is usually insufflation of the stomach with air and subsequent massive regurgitation.
- Inflating the stomach can also splint the diaphragm, making ventilation of the lungs even more difficult.
- Massive inflation of the stomach can result in a vagotonic response and bradycardia.
- Failing to leave sufficient time for expiration and a respiratory pause can cause air trapping in the lungs (autoPEEP) – worsening over inflation found in some acute asthmatic and COPD patients.

Top tips

- Remember we take about 12 breaths a minute. The easiest way to deliver a suitable number of breaths is to squeeze the bag each time you breathe.

- An average adult tidal volume is 500–700 mL. The bag you are using is 1300 mL, so it does not need to be emptied with each breath.
- Inspiration is a smooth and steady process, with expiration twice as long as inspiration. There is a natural post-expiration pause before the next breath begins. Deliver your breaths carefully; they need not be big or fast.
- Leaving dentures in edentulous patients can help give the face structure and make BMV easier, so long as they are well fitting and securely fastened.

- Try using a paediatric size face mask for edentulous patients as the absence of teeth and loss of bone make the point of contact for the mask on the face smaller.
- If there is a leak, listen and place pressure to the side it is heard from. Alternatively, ask an assistant to pull the facial skin gently towards the mask to ensure a snugly fitting facemask with a good seal.

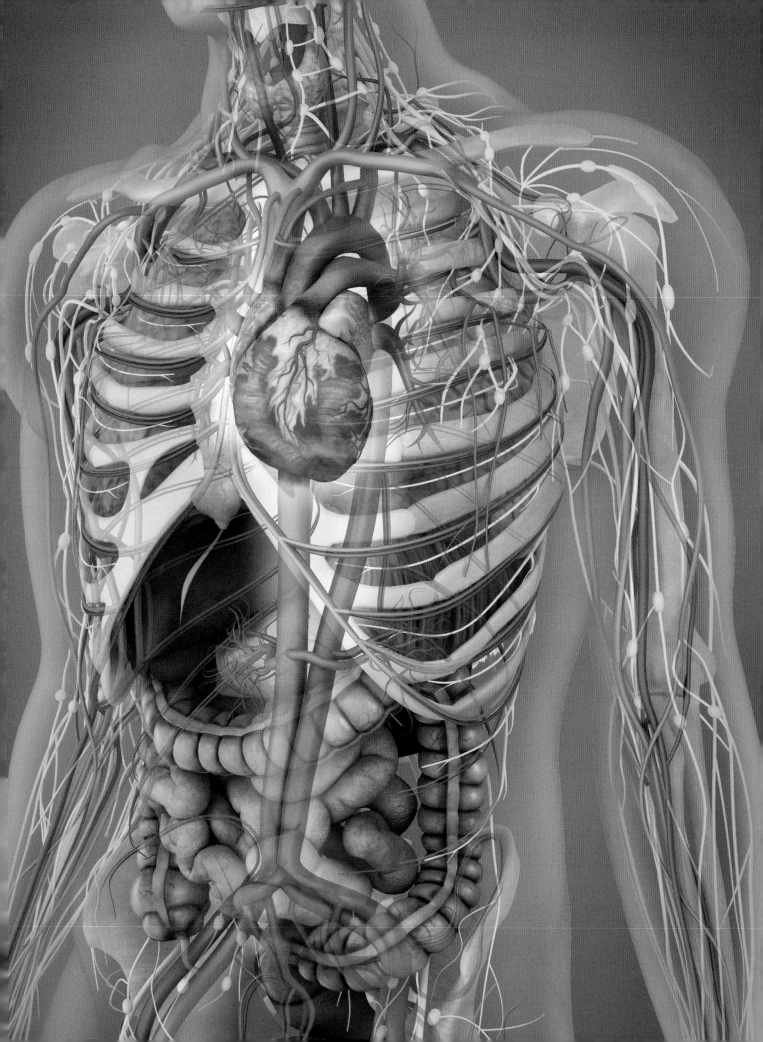

34 Endotracheal intubation (adults)

Jane Sturgess

Figure 34.1 Equipment.

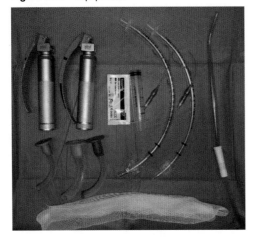

Figure 34.2 'Sniffing the morning air' position.

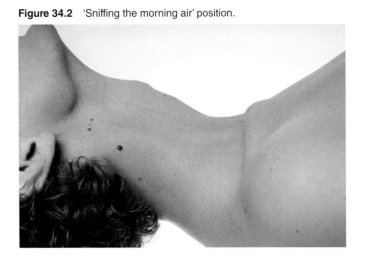

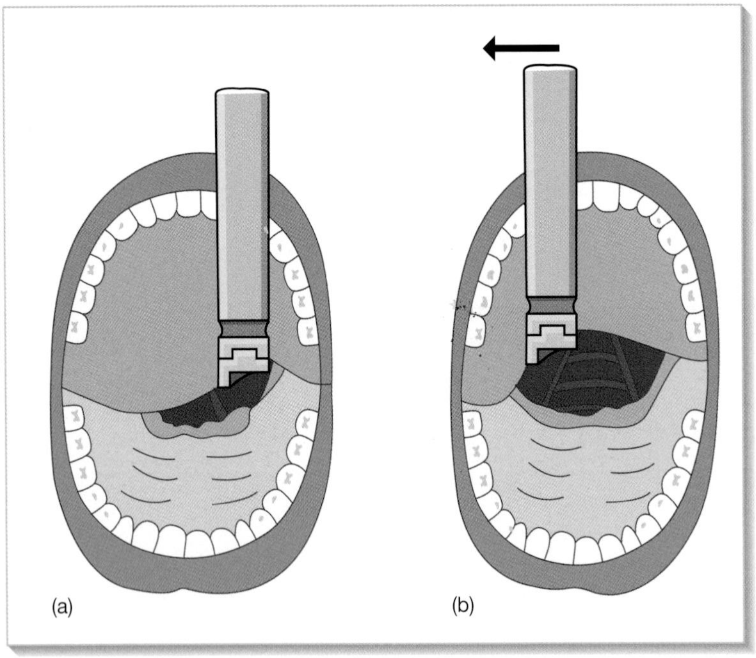

Figure 34.3 Introduction of the laryngoscope blade and sweeping of the tongue to one side, as indicated by arrow.

(a) (b)

Figure 34.4 Correct placement of the laryngoscope blade tip in the vallecula.

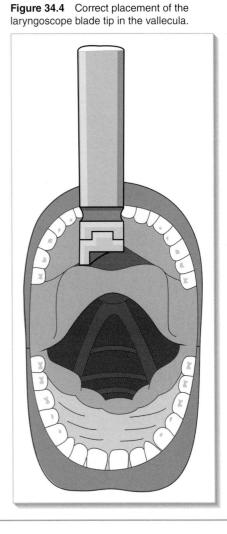

Applied Anatomy for Clinical Procedures at a Glance, First Edition. Jane Sturgess, Francesca Crawley, Ramez Kirollos, and Kirsty Cattle.
© 2021 John Wiley & Sons Ltd. Published 2021 by John Wiley & Sons Ltd.

Figure 34.5 Diagram to show tissue displacement with elevation vs. levering of the laryngoscope blade.

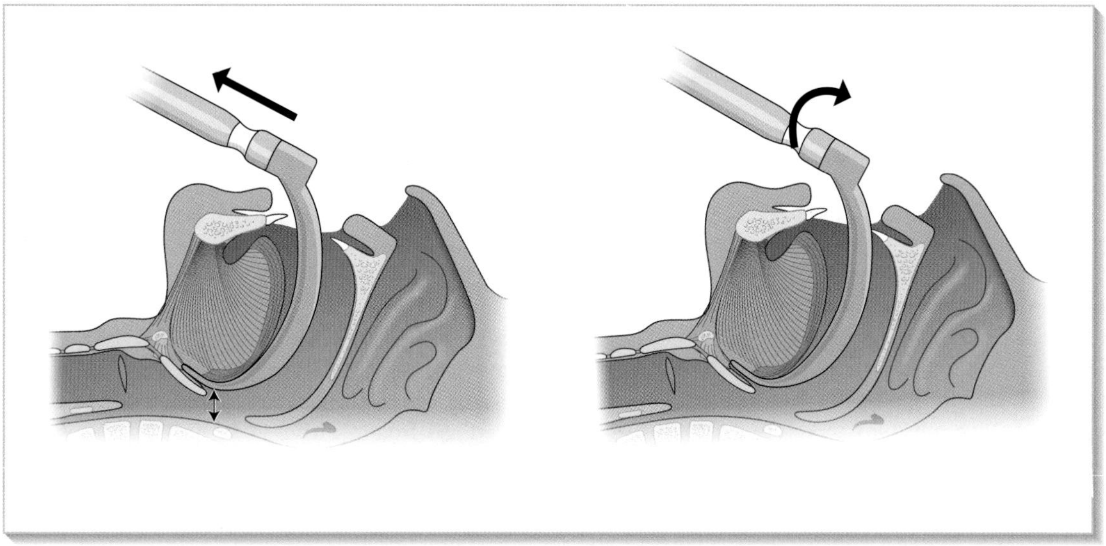

Figure 34.6 The laryngeal inlet.

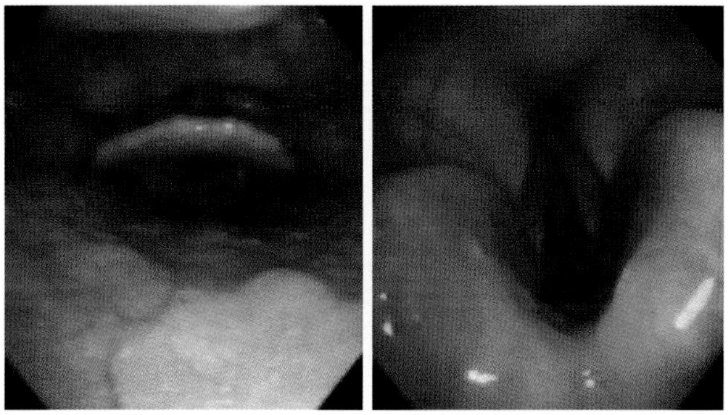

Equipment (Figure 34.1)

As for bag mask ventilation (Chapter 33)

- 2 laryngoscope handles, x2 size C batteries
- Laryngoscope (Macintosh) blade size 3 ♀ and 4 ♂
- Lubricating jelly
- Supraglottic airway size 3, 4, and 5
- Suction and spare Yankauer catheter
- Cuffed endotracheal tube size 7 ♀ and 8 ♂, tube tie, 20 mL syringe filled with air

Technique

This should only ever be performed under direct supervision (by an experienced practitioner). Patients with C-spine injury are not suitable candidates for the inexperienced.

1. Check the lumen of the endotracheal tube (ETT) is patent. Inflate the cuff on the ETT to check its integrity, then deflate it. Lubricate the outer surface of the cuff.
2. In the non-arrested patient an anaesthetic and muscle paralysing agent will be required; these are given by the anaesthetist (or ED physician). Monitor the electrocardiogram, blood pressure, and oxygen saturation (SaO_2).
3. Pre-oxygenate the patient (15 l/min O_2 via a tight fitting mask) either for 3 minutes or with 3 vital capacity breaths.
4. When anaesthetised and paralysed place the head in the 'sniffing the morning air' position, with the neck flexed and the head extended (Figure 34.2).
5. Open the mouth with your right hand and hold the laryngoscope in your left hand. Gently introduce the laryngoscope to the right side of the mouth sweeping the tongue to the left (Figure 34.3).
6. Keep advancing the tip of the laryngoscope until you see the epiglottis. Aim to get the tip of the blade seated well in to the vallecula (Figures 34.4 and 34.5).
7. Lift the blade (and therefore the tongue and epiglottis) upwards and caudad. Do not perform a levering movement – you will break the teeth and still not see the laryngeal inlet. (Figure 34.5)
8. Once you see the glottis (Figure 34.6), take the ETT in your right hand and gently pass it through the cords, making sure one black line marker is below and one above. If there are no markers, place ETT 20 cm at the teeth. Whilst holding the ETT in place gently remove the laryngoscope and inflate the cuff with 5 mL air.
9. Attach the breathing circuit and CO_2 monitor. Insufflate the lungs and check for expired CO_2 and breath sounds in both axillae to confirm endotracheal placement.
10. Check for an audible air leak and add more air to the cuff as necessary. Secure the ETT with the tie and continue manual ventilation, sedation, and paralysis.

Aftercare

- Anaesthesia or sedation and paralysis should be continued whilst the patient is intubated.
- Expired CO_2 should be measured continuously.

- The cuff should be inflated with the least amount of air possible to prevent an air leak. This will reduce the pressure on the tracheal mucosa and reduce the possibility of tracheal stenosis as a late complication.

Common anatomical pitfalls

- Placing the laryngoscope in the midline lets the tongue bulge either side of the blade, obscuring the view of the glottis.
- Movement of the epiglottis to expose the laryngeal inlet depends upon traction on the hypoepiglottic ligament; failing to advance the tip of the laryngoscope blade into the vallecula will result in limited epiglottic displacement.
- Using a levering action to lift the epiglottis only places you at risk of causing dental damage, with the potential to complicate your intubation with a foreign body (tooth!) in the airway. It will also make passing your tube more difficult as it has to manoeuvre an acute angle rather than passing straight into the trachea (Figure 34.5).
- It is important to use the correct size of tube. At times the laryngeal inlet is easily visualised but the ETT will not pass as the tracheal diameter is too small, be prepared to downsize your ETT quickly. Do not force a tube into the trachea – this risks damage (or even perforation) of the tracheal mucosa.

Top tips

- Potential difficult intubation can often be predicted – look out for obesity, beards, small mandibles, prominent front teeth, limited mouth opening, limited neck flexion.
- Head position is crucial – it brings the glottis in line with the posterior border of the tongue and makes visualisation easier. Make sure you have two pillows available and position the head carefully before inserting the laryngoscope.
- Patients with a full stomach or acute abdomen require a 'rapid sequence induction and cricoid pressure' to prevent aspiration of gastric contents.
- The laryngeal inlet may not be in the midline. If you cannot see it straight away and SaO$_2$ >96%, stand a little further back and look to the left in your field of view. Placing gentle **b**ackwards **u**pwards **r**ightwards **p**ressure (BURP) on the thyroid cartilage from the front of the neck may help you visualise the glottis.
- Instead of inserting the ETT in the midline and obscuring your view of the ETT passing through the vocal cords, try starting with the ETT at the right side of the mouth and aiming the tube towards the inlet.

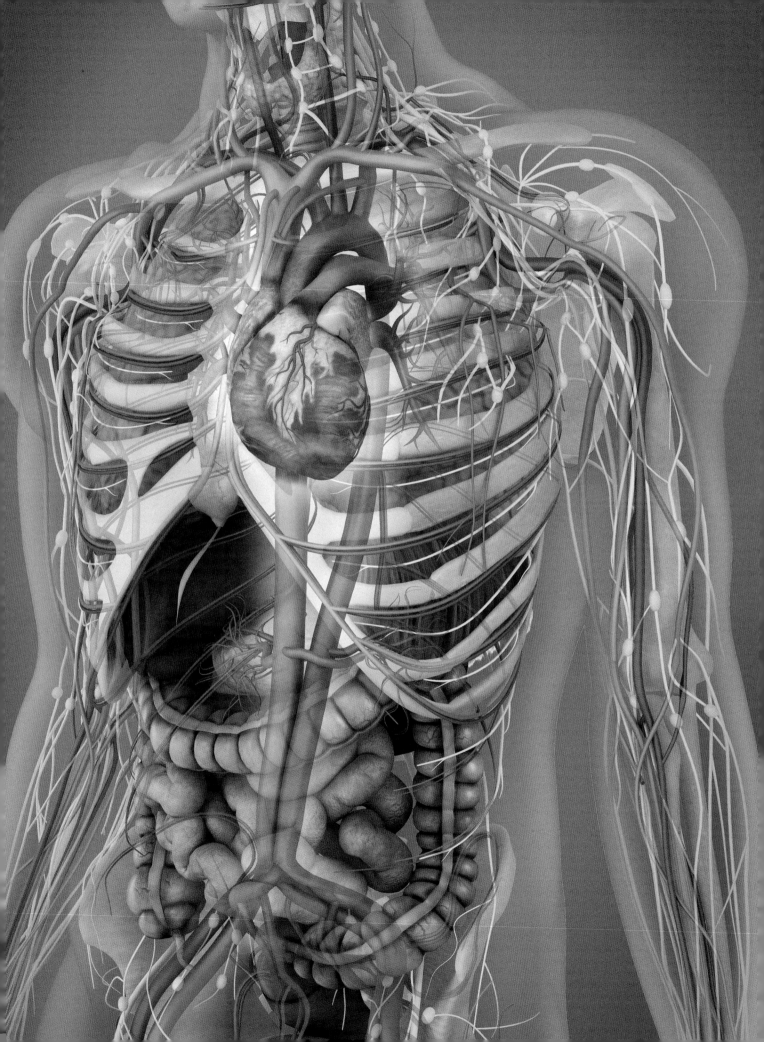

35

Needle cricothryoidotomy (adults)

Jane Sturgess

Figure 35.1 Equipment.

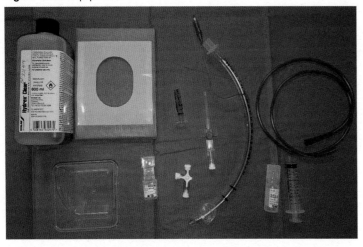

Figure 35.3 (a) Preparing the needle for insertion (b) preparing your trolley with your choice of means of oxygenation.

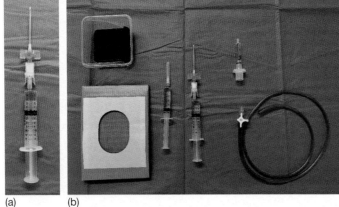

(a)   (b)

Figure 35.4 Patient position and surface anatomy.

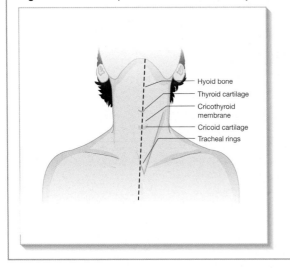

Hyoid bone
Thyroid cartilage
Cricothyroid membrane
Cricoid cartilage
Tracheal rings

Figure 35.2 Ways to ventilate/oxygenate post needle cricothyroidotomy: either (a) with connector from 8 mm endotracheal tube inside a 2 mL syringe, which will connect to a bag valve-mask; or (b) use oxygen tubing and a three-way tap to intermittently oxygenate. It is not possible to ventilate via a needle cricothyroidotomy.

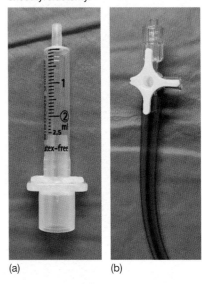

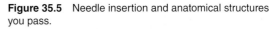

(a)   (b)

Figure 35.5 Needle insertion and anatomical structures you pass.

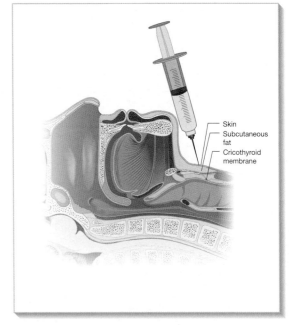

Skin
Subcutaneous fat
Cricothyroid membrane

Applied Anatomy for Clinical Procedures at a Glance, First Edition. Jane Sturgess, Francesca Crawley, Ramez Kirollos, and Kirsty Cattle.
© 2021 John Wiley & Sons Ltd. Published 2021 by John Wiley & Sons Ltd.

Equipment (Figure 35.1)

- Sterile pack and drape, 2% chlorhexidine
- Orange needle
- 5 mL 1% lidocaine
- 2 mL syringe with plunger removed
- Size 8 endotracheal tube 15 mm connector
- Three-way tap
- Full oxygen cylinder, oxygen tubing
- 2x 14 gauge cannula (ideally not a safety cannula)
- 10 mL syringe containing 5 mL saline
- Jet ventilator should be brought to the patient as soon as possible.
  As for bag mask ventilation (Chapter 33) and laryngeal mask airway (Chapter 16)

Technique

Make sure you have called for urgent senior help from anaesthetics and ENT before you start this procedure. This procedure is carried out when you face a patient you cannot intubate or ventilate. They are likely to be cyanosed and distressed, if not unconscious.

It is very stressful; rushing will not help. Take a deep breath and work methodically.

1. Inform the team and patient what you are about to do; you are unlikely to be able to gain proper informed consent. Nonetheless, explaining to the patient or your assistant will give you the opportunity to order your thoughts and mentally prepare yourself for the next steps.
2. Pre-oxygenate the patient with 100% O_2 and give high flow oxygen via a tightly fitting facemask with a rebreathe bag during the procedure. Uncover the anterior chest wall so that you can easily see it rise and fall with ventilation.
3. Prepare the ventilation circuit you will attach to your needle – there are two options: bag mask valve connection or oxygen tubing connection (Figure 35.2).
4. Prepare your cannula for insertion. Remove the bung from the end of the cannula. Attach the 10 mL syringe half-filled with 5 mL saline. Withdraw the plunger to double check that air bubbles are drawn into the syringe and are easily visible (Figure 35.3a).
5. Arrange a sterile trolley at the patients bedside with all your prepared equipment easily to hand and in order of anticipated use (Figure 35.3b).
6. Monitor oxygen saturation (SaO_2), electrocardiogram, and blood pressure. Call for CO_2 monitor.
7. Place the patient supine, extend their neck, and prepare a sterile field across the anterior neck from mental symphysis to the sternal notch and to both posterior borders of sternocleidomastoid.
8. Identify the midline, the hyoid bone, thyroid cartilage, cricoid cartilage, cricothyroid membrane (it is the indented section between the 2 cartilages), and tracheal rings (Figure 35.4).
9. Gently hold the larynx between your nondominant thumb and index finger at the level of the cricithyroid membrane. Pull the skin tight.
10. Feel the cricothyroid membrane again with the tip of your dominant index finger.
11. Take your prepared cannula and syringe in your dominant hand and insert the cannula through the membrane in the midline. Direct the needle towards the feet (caudally) at an angle of 30–45 degrees from the bed (Figure 35.5).

12. Advance the needle through the skin, subcutaneous tissue, and cricothyroid membrane whilst continuously aspirating the syringe plunger, looking for bubbles to appear in the saline. Bubbles confirm intratracheal placement.
13. Advance the cannula and needle a couple of mm further, then advance the cannula to the hub whilst holding the needle in place. Remove the needle and detach the syringe.
14. Connect the syringe to the cannula and aspirate checking for bubbles. Always keep hold of the cannula and check it doesn't kink/obstruct.
15. If bubbles are present attach your ventilation circuit and gently inflate the lungs whilst watching for the chest to rise. Stop if the neck swells.
16. Consider siting a second cannula to allow passage of expired gases if the airway is completely obstructed. Leave it open to air.
17. Resite the needle if the neck swells or no air is aspirated.
18. Oxygenate the patient by connecting to an oxygen source for a count of 1 second and opening to air (to allow 'expiration') for a count of 4 seconds.

Aftercare

- Continuously ensure the cannula is in the trachea.
- Observe for barotrauma.
- Arrange for definitive airway (often surgical).
- Contact intensive therapy unit.
- Start diagnosis and treatment of the cause of airway obstruction.

Common anatomical pitfalls

- Failure of expiration – this is due to an obstructed upper airway. Even once the needle cricothyroidotomy has been placed, efforts must continue to open the airway to permit expiration and avoid baro- and volutrauma to the lungs. Look for and treat pneumothorax.
- Surgical emphysema – ventilation into the soft tissues of the anterior triangle of the neck via a displaced cannula can cause rapid and massive surgical emphysema, with irretrievable airway obstruction, as air travels through the fascial plains of the neck in a circumferential fashion.
- Tracheal ring damage – cannula inserted too low and directly into the trachea. Oxygenation will still be possible as is a surgical airway but the tracheostomy cuff may get torn by the fractured tracheal ring during insertion.
- Posterior tracheal wall damage – the needle is advanced too far. This can potentially lead to pneumomediastinum.
- Haemorrhage – this can be from the superior laryngeal artery (from the superior thyroid branch of the internal carotid) as it enters the larynx through the lateral aperture of the thyrohyoid membrane if the needle insertion is too high, or from the vessels found in the carotid sheath (common and internal carotid, internal jugular) if the needle is inserted too laterally.
- Nerve damage to the external laryngeal nerve, which supplies the cricothyroid membrane (derived from the superior laryngeal nerve arising from the inferior ganglia of the vagus nerve and a branch of the superior cervical sympathetic ganglion). The recurrent laryngeal nerves (branches of the vagus) supply sensory innervation to the larynx below the vocal cords, and motor supply to all laryngeal muscles bar the cricothyroid membrane. The vagus nerve can be damaged if the carotid sheath is punctured.

Top tips

- Contraindications are laryngeal injury, tracheal rupture, laryngotracheal disruption.
- Needle cricothyroidotomy may be very useful when the epiglottis causes partial airway obstruction on inspiration (e.g. epiglottitis causing a 'ball-valve' effect), as expiration will be normal.
- Watch the chest rise and fall with jet ventilation. If there is limited fall of the chest the upper airway is still obstructed and the lungs are at risk of baro-/volutrauma. Increase the expiratory time, and check for pneumothorax.
- Keeping in the midline minimises complications from damage of neurovascular structures. The cricothyroid membrane in the midline is only covered by skin and subcutaneous tissue (and median cricothyroid ligament) with occasional anastomosis between both cricothyroid arteries or branches of inferior thyroid vein and may cause minor haemorrhage. On either side it is covered by the paired cricothyroid muscles underlying the medial edges of the sternohyoids. The major neurovascular structures such as the carotid sheath, superior thyroid arteries, and recurrent laryngeal nerves are laterally placed in relationship to the larynx and trachea.

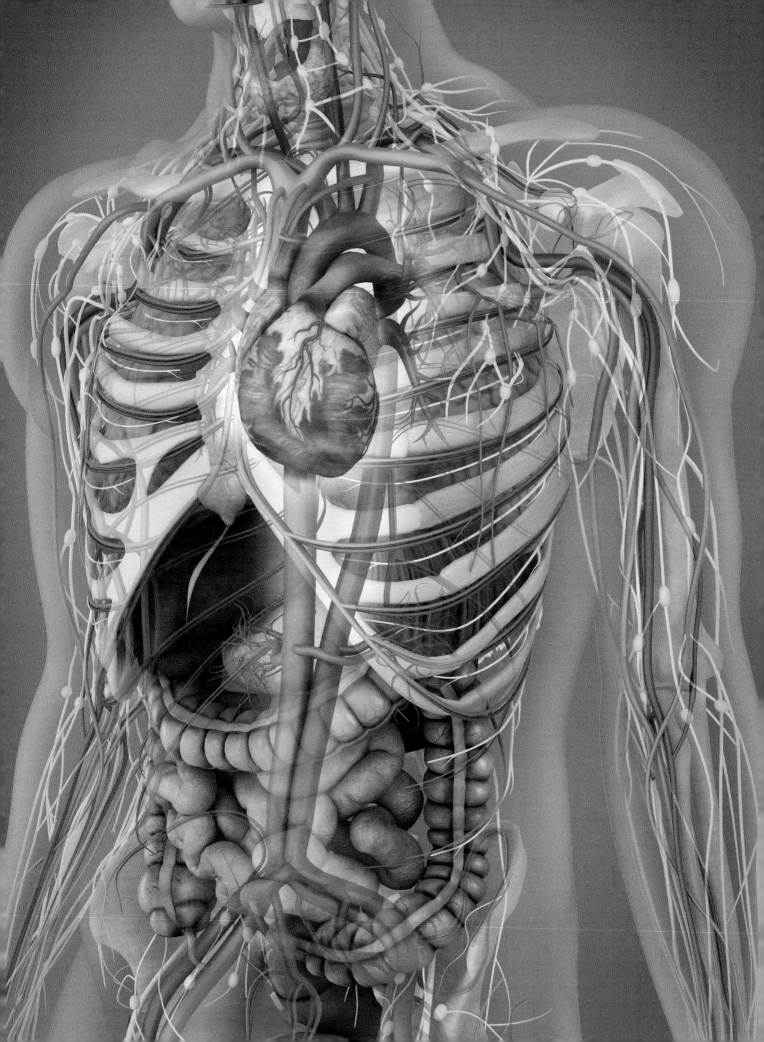

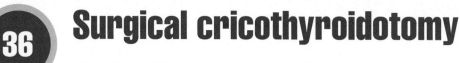

Surgical cricothyroidotomy

36

Sherif Kirollos and Ramez Kirollos

Figure 36.1   Anterior neck surface anatomy and interior anatomy.

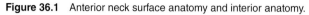
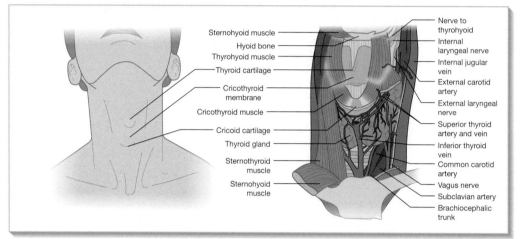

Figure 36.2   Procedure. After locating and stabilising the cricothyroid membrane, make a transverse incision down through the cricothyroid membrane (a). Dilate the incision up (b-c) then place the tracheostomy tube through the incision and inflate the balloon (d).

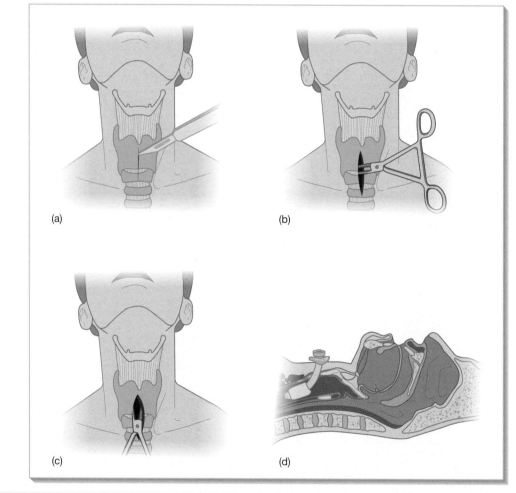

Applied Anatomy for Clinical Procedures at a Glance, First Edition. Jane Sturgess, Francesca Crawley, Ramez Kirollos, and Kirsty Cattle.

Equipment

- Sterile gloves, gown, face shield
- Antiseptic solution for skin preparation such as chlorhexidine or povidone-iodine
- Fenestrated sterile towel
- Gauze
- Local anaesthetic
- Syringe with 18–21 gauge needle
- Tracheostomy tube (6mm internal diameter) or endotracheal tube
- Scalpel with number 11 blade
- Trousseau dilator
- Curved haemostat
- Suture
- Tracheal hook
- Sterile dressing

Indications

- Inability to intubate and ventilate
- Local airway trauma or obstruction

Contraindications

- Massive trauma to larynx or cricoid cartilage
- Orotracheal and nasotracheal intubation not yet attempted
- Not recommended in children below 10 years of age as more liable to post-procedural traumatic sequelae

Procedure (Figure 36.2)

1. Check your equipment.
2. Position the patient in a supine position with neck in extension. Avoid excessive neck manipulations if cervical-spine injury is suspected but securing the airway is the priority.
3. If time permits, clean the site with antiseptic solution.
4. Administer local anaesthetic.
5. Stabilise the larynx and locate the thyroid cartilage via palpation. From here, palpate inferiorly to locate the cricoid cartilage. The cricothyroid membrane is situated between the cricoid cartilage and thyroid cartilage, where the incision will be made (Figure 36.1).
6. Make a 2.5 cm vertical incision through the subcutaneous tissue overlying the cricothyroid membrane. Creating a vertical incision avoids damage to the recurrent laryngeal nerves situated on either side of the trachea.
7. Make a blunt dissection using a curved haemostat. Extend the incision if necessary.
8. Using a size 10 or 11 blade, create a horizontal incision through the cricothyroid membrane.
9. Entering the trachea will be confirmed through audible airflow.
10. With the blade remaining within the trachea, insert the trachea hook and catch the distal site of the incision and retract anteriorly, elevating the larynx. Remove the blade once the hook is in place.
11. Open the membrane vertically using a trousseau dilator.
12. Insert the tracheotomy tube, inflate the cuff, and secure it.
13. Connect the tube to a ventilator.
14. Check for a symmetrical rise of the chest wall and auscultate for breath sounds.

Aftercare

- Request a chest X-ray to confirm the position of tracheostomy tube
- The tube through the cricothyroidotomy can be left up to 72 hours. If ventilation is needed beyond this, it should be converted to tracheostomy.

Common anatomical pitfalls

- Making the horizontal incision too deep can penetrate the posterior laryngeal wall and subsequently the oesophagus.
- Complications include oesophageal perforation, subcutaneous emphysema often caused by the horizontal incision being made too wide, bleeding or haemorrhage through vessel rupture. Smaller vessel bleeding can often be controlled through pressure, whereas bleeding from major vessels such as the common carotid arteries or internal jugular vein may require ligation.

Top tip

- A midline vertical incision has an advantage over a horizontal incision in cases in which the landmarks are not easily palpable.

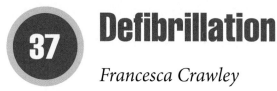

Defibrillation

Francesca Crawley

Figure 37.1 Equipment.

Figure 37.2 Defibrillator pad positions.

Figure 37.3 Cardiac action potential and the contribution of different parts of the heart to the ECG trace.

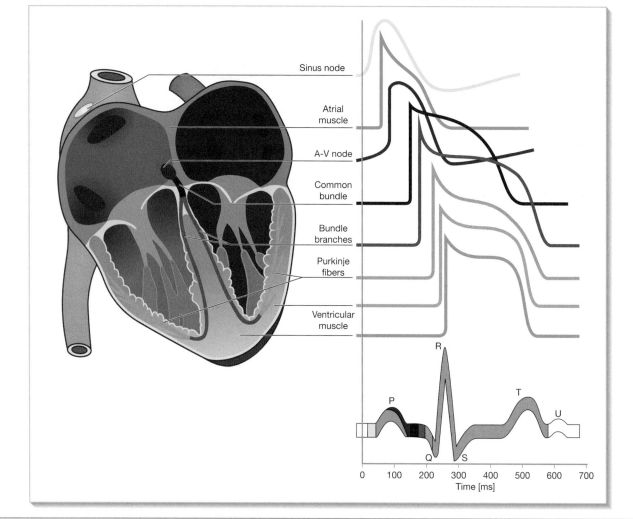

Sinus node

Atrial muscle

A-V node

Common bundle

Bundle branches

Purkinje fibers

Ventricular muscle

R

P

T

U

Q   S

Time [ms]

0   100   200   300   400   500   600   700

Applied Anatomy for Clinical Procedures at a Glance, First Edition. Jane Sturgess, Francesca Crawley, Ramez Kirollos, and Kirsty Cattle.

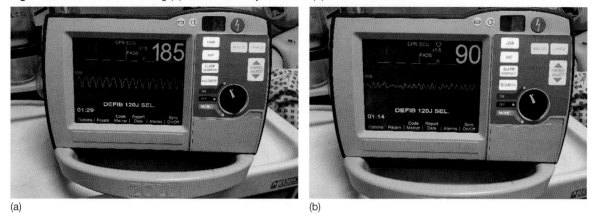

Figure 37.4 Defibrillator showing (a) ventricular tachycardia and (b) ventricular fibrillation.

(a)   (b)

Equipment (Figure 37.1)

- Defibrillator – check if it is monophasic or biphasic
- Defibrillator pads x 2
- Electrocardiogram (ECG) 'dots' and ECG leads
- Cardiac arrest trolley
- Cardiac arrest team
- Ambu Bag and oxygen
- Intravenous cannula
- Intravenous giving set and 1 litre fluid

Technique

1. Expose the whole of the patient's chest, remove vomit or secretions, and make sure the chest wall is dry.
2. Turn the defibrillator on.
3. Ensure the defibrillator pads are connected to leads. Connect the pad leads to the defibrillator.
4. Place the cardiac apex pad over the 5th intercostal space in the midaxillary line, with the long axis of the pad in line with the intercostal space (Figure 37.2). The entire pad should be firmly adherent to the patient's skin; any other monitoring lines should be placed as far away from the pad as possible.
5. Place the second pad along the right sternal edge, with the long axis of the pad parallel to the long axis of the sternum (Figure 37.2). Pad position is important to ensure the energy is delivered through the maximum volume of cardiac muscle, along the conduction pathways.
6. Check the rhythm. This is done automatically with an automated external defibrillator (AED). Confirm the patient is in ventricular fibrillation (VF) or pulseless ventricular tachycardia (VT) (Figure 37.4).
7. Choose your energy for defibrillation – 360 Joules monophasic, 120–200 Joules biphasic.
8. Ask the team to stand clear.
9. Check that team members are standing away from the patient and that neither they nor equipment they are holding are touching the patient.
10. Charge your defibrillator and state loudly and clearly 'Stand clear, charging'.
11. Perform a last quick check that all members are clear and administer the shock. State loudly and clearly 'Stand clear, shocking'.
12. Recommence CPR according to advanced cardiovascular life support guidelines.

Aftercare

- In patients with return of spontaneous circulation observe the respiratory effort and support breathing as necessary.
- Continuously monitor the ECG and keep the pads attached to the patient.
- Place the patient in the recovery position to protect the airway.
- Consider where the patient should be cared for and help the team arrange this; the patient will often be transferred to coronary care or intensive care.
- Be prepared to request a chest X-ray or perform arterial blood gas sampling.

Common anatomical pitfalls

- Remember that the right ventricle sits anteriorly under the left sternal border, with the left ventricle more posteriorly. The anatomical position of the healthy left ventricular apex is the 4th intercostal space, anterior axillary line. The apex beat is displaced inferolaterally in dilated cardiomyopathy, sometimes to the 6th intercostal space, midaxillary line. The position of defibrillation pads takes the ventricular positions in health and disease into account.
- Remember the normal pathway for electrical conduction through the heart, from the sinoatrial node in the right atrium at the insertion of the superior vena cava, to the atrioventricular node situated at the junction of the atria and the ventricles, along the bundle of His (in the interventricular septum), before it divides into the right and left bundle that supply their respective ventricles. The fibres run close to the ventricular cavities and send sub-branches (Purkinje fibres) through the bulk of the ventricular muscle. The aim of defibrillation is to override any aberrant electrical activity, allowing the heart to reset to normal rhythm. Selecting the correct energy is important (Figure 37.3).
- Obese subjects have a large amount of subcutaneous tissue that can absorb energy delivered. This is called raised impedance. Choosing a higher initial energy can reduce this problem.
- Any substance that comes between the surface of the pad and the patient's skin can cause a failure in delivery of energy to the heart – hair, piercings. A large gap can cause electrical arcing and burns. In addition a poorly applied pad can cause very dense current delivery (and electrical burns) in areas of contact.

Top tips

- Alternative pad positions are anteroposterior, with the pads placed at the right sternal edge, and between the tip of the left scapula and the spinous processes of the upper thoracic spine. This is useful in patients with implantable electronic devices (pacemaker/deep brain stimulator).

- Monophasic machines deliver charge in one direction only, whereas biphasic defibrillators deliver the charge first in one direction, and then in the electrically opposite direction. Energy travels from the sternal to the apical and then back to the sternal pad. Biphasic defibrillators deliver more consistent current and terminate more arrhythmias (and at lower energies) than monophasic defibrillators.

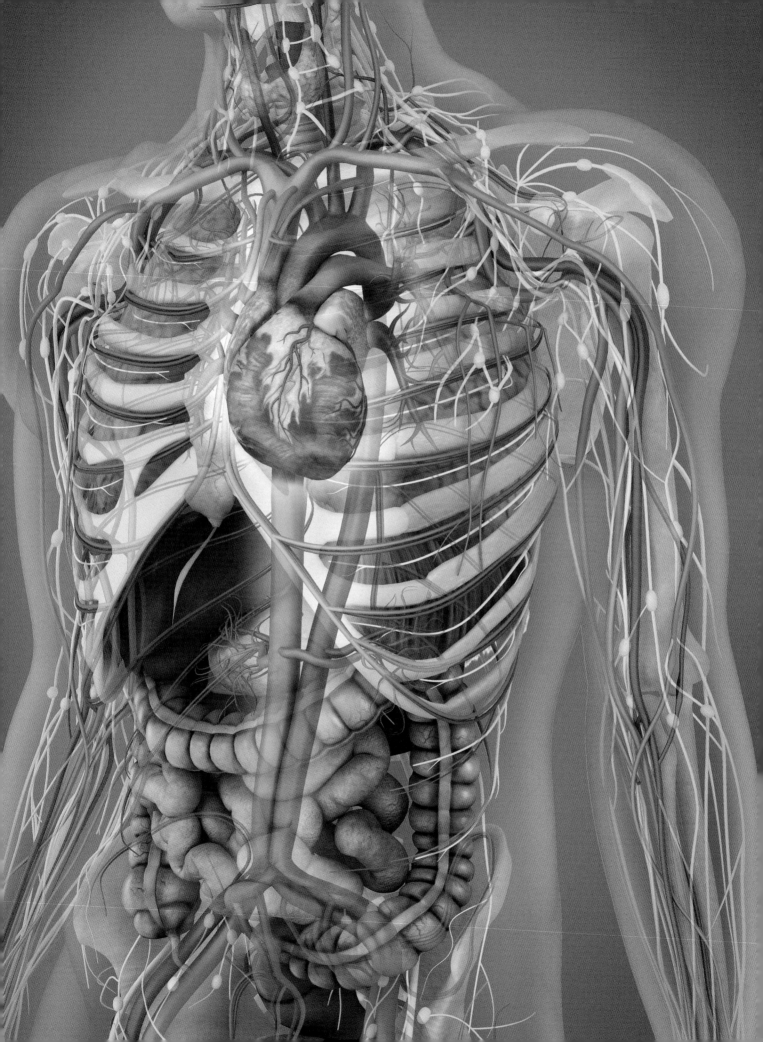

38 Spinal injection

Jane Sturgess

Figure 38.1 Equipment.

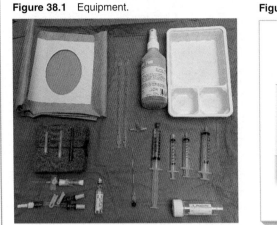

Figure 38.2 Patient position and surface anatomy.

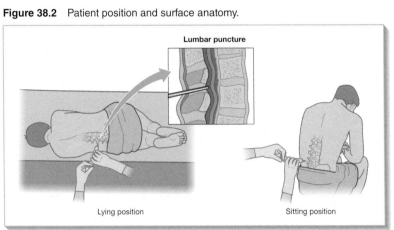

Lumbar puncture

Lying position

Sitting position

Figure 38.3 Needle direction and sagittal anatomy.

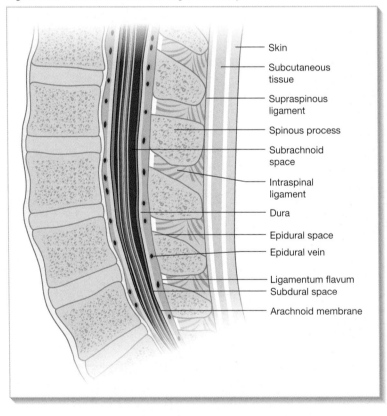

- Skin
- Subcutaneous tissue
- Supraspinous ligament
- Spinous process
- Subrachnoid space
- Intraspinal ligament
- Dura
- Epidural space
- Epidural vein
- Ligamentum flavum
- Subdural space
- Arachnoid membrane

Applied Anatomy for Clinical Procedures at a Glance, First Edition. Jane Sturgess, Francesca Crawley, Ramez Kirollos, and Kirsty Cattle.
© 2021 John Wiley & Sons Ltd. Published 2021 by John Wiley & Sons Ltd.

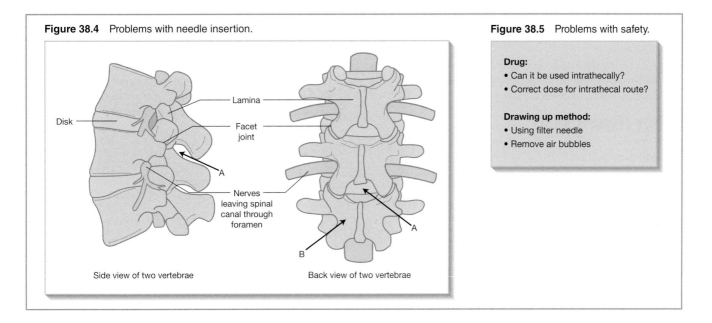

Figure 38.4 Problems with needle insertion.

Labels on figure:
- Disk
- Lamina
- Facet joint
- Nerves leaving spinal canal through foramen
- A
- B
- Side view of two vertebrae
- Back view of two vertebrae

Figure 38.5 Problems with safety.

Drug:
- Can it be used intrathecally?
- Correct dose for intrathecal route?

Drawing up method:
- Using filter needle
- Remove air bubbles

Equipment (Figure 38.1)

See also Scrubbing up (Chapter 1), Sterile field (Chapter 2), Local anaesthetic (Chapter 5).
- 25 gauge and 23 gauge needle
- 1 mL, 2 mL, and 5 mL syringe
- 5–10 mL 1% lidocaine
- Spinal needle 25 gauge or 22 gauge
- Injectate – usually 0.5% bupivacaine +/- opiate, or chemotherapy

Technique

1. Establish IV access and monitor oxygen saturation (SaO$_2$), electrocardiogram (ECG), and blood pressure.
2. **Position** the patient in the left lateral position with their back parallel to the edge of the bed, the knees and hips flexed as far as possible and the head and neck flexed (see Figure 38.2), or alternatively have the patient sitting, with their feet supported on a stool to flex the patient at their hips and knees, ask them to 'hug a pillow and put their chin onto their chest'. These positions decrease the lumbar lordosis and open the interspinous space.
3. **Identify the L4/5 interspinous space** (see Figure 24.3).
4. Feel for the highest point of both iliac crests.
5. Draw (or imagine) a line between these points. This is called Tuffier's line and marks either the spinous process of L4 or the L4/5 interspinous space.
6. The lower aspects of the 10th rib correspond to the L1/2 interspace – a useful landmark in the obese patient.
7. It can be useful to mark the spaces above and below.
8. **Prepare a sterile field**, scrub and anaesthetise the tissues (warn the patient that the skin preparation is cold and the local anaesthetic stings).
9. Using a 25 gauge needle raise a skin wheal with up to 1 mL 1% lidocaine.
10. Insert a 20 gauge needle through the centre of the wheal to the hilt and use 5–10 mL 1% lidocaine to anaesthetise the deeper tissues as the needle is withdrawn towards the skin, aspirating before injecting.
11. Repeat this process in a couple of slightly different directions to ensure all tissue is numb.
12. This will allow you to get a 'feel' for the direction and depth you should aim for with the spinal needle.
13. Whilst waiting for the local anaesthetic to work **prepare your equipment** so that it is easy to get exactly what you want. Draw up your desired drug (s) to inject.
14. **Insertion of the needle**. Remember the direction of the spinous processes and aim slightly cephalad (Figure 38.3).
15. Advance slowly and steadily. The needle passes through skin, subcutaneous fat, supraspinous ligament, interspinous ligament, ligamentum flavum, and finally dura. Your needle will be firmly gripped by the tissues when it sits in the interspinous ligament. You should feel a characteristic 'pop' as the dura is breached and cerebrospinal fluid (CSF) should flow. This is commonly at 4–5 cm.
16. Connect your prepared syringe of injectate to the spinal needle. Consider gently aspirating CSF into the syringe to confirm intrathecal placement and free flow of CSF before injecting your prepared mixture/drug.
17. Remove the needle (and introducer needle) in a single movement and apply gently pressure to the needle puncture site (especially if it is bleeding).
18. A small plaster or sterile spray can suffice as a dressing.
19. Place the patient supine and continue to monitor SaO$_2$, ECG, and BP. The patient can become hypotensive in response to the chemical sympathectomy induced by anaesthetising the lumbosacral sympathetic outflow if local anaesthetic is used.

Aftercare

As for post-lumbar puncture (Chapter 24)
- Monitor for prolonged effects of the injectate, specifically return of motor function following spinal anaesthesia.

Common anatomical pitfalls

As for lumbar puncture – Chapter 24

Top tips

As for lumbar puncture (Chapter 24). See also Figure 38.4.

Difficulty aspirating CSF

- Either low CSF pressure or collapse of thecal sack due to negative pressure generated as the plunger on the syringe is withdrawn. Use a smaller volume syringe to create less negative pressure.

- The lumen of the needle has become obstructed either with softy tissue or clot. Gently inject 0.2–0.4 mL saline and check for CSF flow.
- The lumen of the needle has moved – check that CSF flows from the open end of the spinal needle after removing the syringe. Reposition the needle if required.

Safety (Figure 38.5)

- Always check the drug you are delivering (and its diluent) is safe to use intrathecally.

- Draw up drugs from glass ampoules with a filter needle to reduce your risk of injecting particulate matter.
- Always check the dose of drug you are administering is at the appropriate concentration and dilution.
- Always remove air bubbles from the syringe that contains your injectate. Whilst an air bubble is unlikely to cause a systemic circulatory collapse, it can cause a severe headache and back pain.

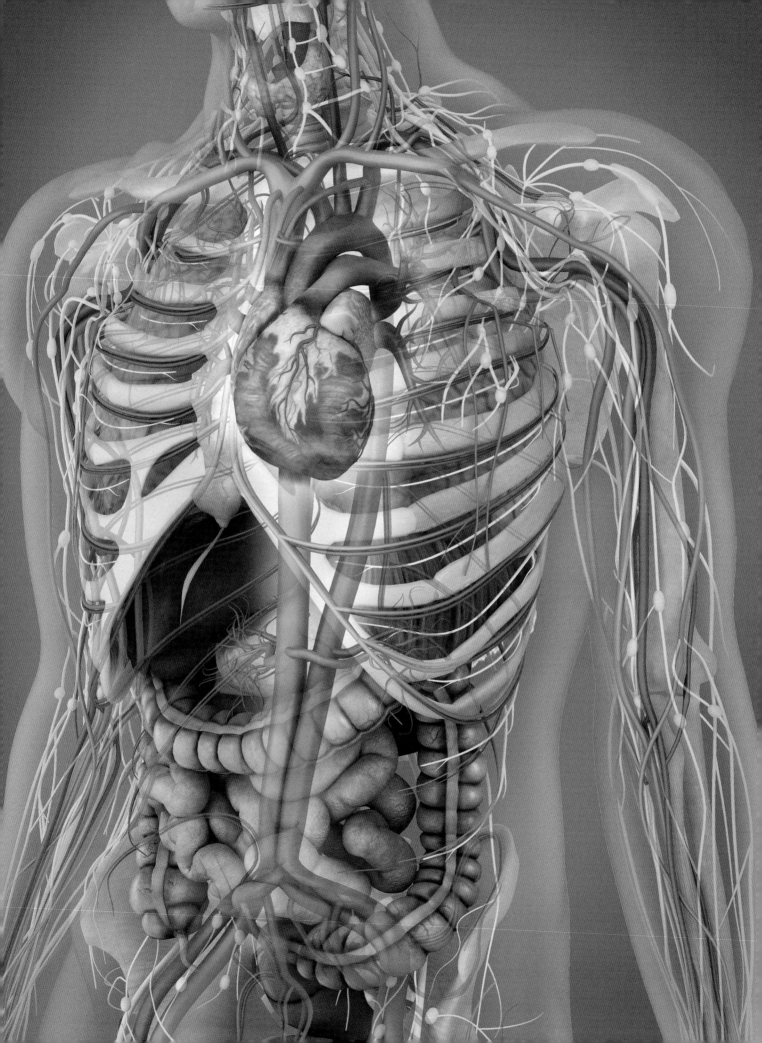

Epidural injection

Jane Sturgess

Figure 39.1 Equipment.

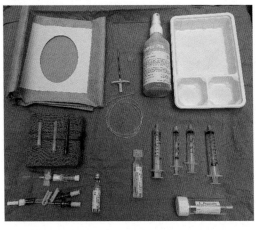

Figure 39.2 Features of the epidural needle (a) and catheter (b).

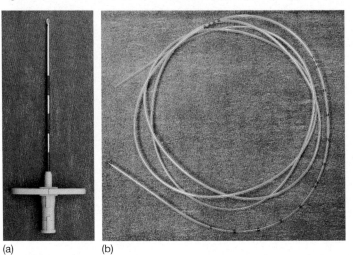

(a)   (b)

Figure 39.3 Continuous loss of resistance.

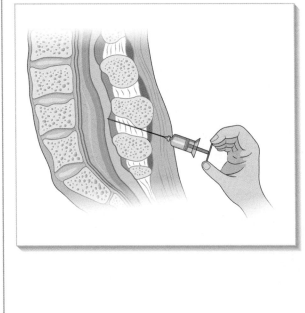

Figure 39.4 Sagittal section to show the anatomical structures the needle passes and the epidural space as it 'opens' – the needle stops advancing and the plunger on the syringe depresses as the space fills with saline (or air).

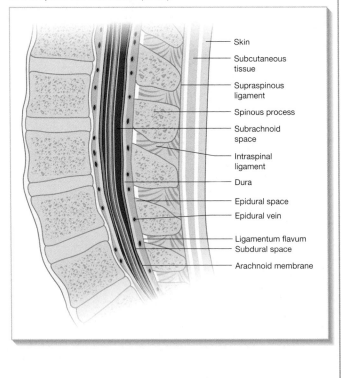

Skin
Subcutaneous tissue
Supraspinous ligament
Spinous process
Subrachnoid space
Intraspinal ligament
Dura
Epidural space
Epidural vein
Ligamentum flavum
Subdural space
Arachnoid membrane

Applied Anatomy for Clinical Procedures at a Glance, First Edition. Jane Sturgess, Francesca Crawley, Ramez Kirollos, and Kirsty Cattle.
© 2021 John Wiley & Sons Ltd. Published 2021 by John Wiley & Sons Ltd.

Equipment (Figure 39.1)

Also see the following chapters: Scrubbing up (Chapter 1), Sterile field (Chapter 2), Local anaesthetic (Chapter 5).
- 25 gauge and 23 gauge needle
- 2 mL and 5 mL syringe
- 5 mL 1% lidocaine
- Saline 10 mL
- Epidural needle
- Epidural pack

Technique

1. Follow steps 1–13 for spinal injection (Chapter 38).
2. Check that the epidural catheter passes freely through the introducer and the epidural needle.
3. Connect the epidural filter to the catheter and flush with saline to check the catheter is patent and that the fluid exits the three holes (distal, medial, and proximal).
4. Replace the stylet into the epidural needle, make sure the bed is at a comfortable height and sit down facing the patient's back.
5. Note that the epidural needle has markings along its length to permit you to calculate the distance to its tip (Figure 39.2b).
6. The epidural needle is blunter than the standard Quinke (cutting bevel) tip needle. It will need persistent pressure to break through the skin at first. Be careful to control the depth of initial needle insertion.
7. Follow steps 16 and 17 for spinal injection. Once your epidural needle is in the intraspinous ligament (about 2–3 cm; Figure 39.4) it will become firmly gripped by the tissues. If you let go of the needle it will maintain its position and direction. Remove the stylet and connect the 5 mL saline filled syringe to the epidural needle.
8. To use a continuous loss of resistance to saline technique it is now important to change from advancing the epidural needle with direct manipulation of the needle to indirect pressure from the syringe plunger to advance the needle tip (Figure 39.3).
9. Consider the syringe of saline and the epidural needle as a single unit.
10. Resistance of the interspinous ligament and the ligamentum flavum is high, with ligamentum flavum higher than interspinous ligament.
11. Pressure on the plunger in the face of high pressure at the needle tip will result in the unit moving forwards as one, with advancement of the epidural needle tip through the interspinous ligament and ligamentum flavum.
12. The epidural space is found immediately anterior to the ligamentum flavum. Importantly it is a potential space. When the tip of the epidural needle breaches the ligamentum flavum and enters the epidural space the pressure resistance at the tip of the needle immediately drops, whilst pressure on the syringe plunger remains constant.
13. The unit stops moving forward but the plunger of the syringe depresses and saline is injected into the epidural space, opening it up.
14. Note the depth of the needle tip from the skin by counting the marks that can still be seen on the needle. This is the depth of the epidural space. It is usually about 5 cm.
15. Gently aspirate the syringe to check for blood.
16. Disconnect the syringe to check for cerebrospinal fluid (CSF). A few drops of saline at this point are common. CSF leak produces a continuous flow of fluid.
17. For single shot therapeutic epidural injections, connect the syringe with your injectate making sure there are no air bubbles, gently aspirate again, then administer your injection. Remove the needle and syringe as a single unit.
18. To site an epidural catheter, connect the introducer (if you choose to use it). Insert the catheter, with the coloured distal tip first, into the needle and gently advance. The length of the needle and introducer is 10 cm. Warn the patient when the catheter is at 10 cm that they may experience an 'odd' sensation in their back but that it should be short lived. Advance the catheter further. Remember you will want to leave 4 cm of catheter inside the epidural space (4 cm+depth of epidural space=length of catheter cm, fixed at the skin)

Aftercare

- Monitor for allergic reactions to the injectate.
- Monitor pulse, blood pressure, oxygen saturation (SaO_2).
- Check for motor block (using the bromage score) and seek help if the motor block is denser than expected.
- Check for severe back pain as a sign of epidural haematoma
- Check the insertion site for blood, CSF, or signs of infection. Any concerns need urgent medical review.
- Check the catheter has been removed in its entirety, including the coloured tip on the end when it is removed.
- Send the tip of the epidural catheter to microbiology for culture after removal to check for infection.

Common anatomical pitfalls

- Off midline – check the needle is passing parallel to the floor and that the bed is flat.
- Bloody tap – off the midline and hitting an epidural vessel. You may need to abandon the procedure.
- Neuralgia whilst finding the epidural space with the needle – ask which leg the pain went to. This means you are off midline. Pain to the left indicates your needle tip is to the left. Withdraw your needle and reinsert 0.5 cm to the right (or away from the floor if you are in the left lateral position)
- CSF – dural tap. Your needle tip has advanced through the epidural space, breeched the dura and your needle tip is now intrathecal. Check the length of your needle tip carefully as you advance.
- CSF – watch post procedure for post-dural puncture headache. Immediate management is bedrest, increase oral fluids and prescribe simple regular analgesics. Oral caffeine may help. Severe cases may require an epidural blood patch, contact the on-call anaesthetist.
- Unresolving neuralgia on insertion of the epidural catheter – your original needle insertion may have been slightly off midline and the tip of the catheter has migrated from the epidural space into the nerve sheath and exited the epidural space along the nerve root.
- Bone only – you are most likely off midline and are hitting successive laminae. Either withdraw your needle and start again in the midline or change the insertion angle of your needle and aim to walk the tip of your needle off the lamina into the midline. The ligamentum flavum is at its thinnest here and you will come to the epidural space very soon after leaving the bone. NB periosteum is supplied by pain fibres. This approach can be painful to the patient and will require extra local anaesthetic.
- Patients with kyphosis or scoliosis. As the spinal column twists the location of the thecal sac behind it becomes less predictable. Ask for senior help.

- Calcified ligamentum flavum in the elderly can make location of the epidural space challenging. Bamboo spine in ankylosing spondylitis can present a similar problem. Horse riders and dancers often have a well-developed ligamentum flavum. Calcified or well-developed ligaments can be confused for bone.
- Arthritis of the lumbar spine can reduce your ability to flex the patient in order to reduce the lumbar lordosis and open up the interspinous space.
- Unilateral blocks can occur – refer to the anaesthetist.

Top tips

- Try sitting the patient if it is difficult to visualise the midline and ask them to point to the middle of their back.
- CSF - You will either need to abandon or, if appropriate, consider changing drug doses and treating as a spinal. This is potentially very unsafe and should be discussed with your senior. Further injections through a spinal catheter should be checked by the doctor.
- More than a few drops of fluid from the needle tip after insertion, or fluid aspirated from the epidural catheter, unsure if it is CSF. Place a drop on a glucostix – CSF will test positive, saline injectate will not.
- Bloody aspirate from epidural catheter – flush with 2 mL saline, disconnect the filter and place the end of the catheter below the skin insertion point. Wait and see if gravity induces blood flow. Epidural vessels are thin walled and collapse easily with the negative pressure induced by withdrawing the plunger on a syringe. Negative aspiration at this point would not necessarily exclude intravascular placement of the tip of the epidural catheter. If no blood flows reattach the filter and gently aspirate the catheter (using a small syringe, e.g. 2 mL). If there is blood you will need to abandon and start again.
- Continuous back pain at the insertion site or excessive motor block that does not resolve should alert you to the potential for an epidural haematoma. This is a neurological emergency. Seek senior help and arrange an MRI to exclude or confirm the diagnosis. The sooner the clot is evacuated the better the neurological recovery.
- Once you are familiar with lumbar epidurals you will progress to thoracic and cervical epidurals. Whilst the loss of resistance to saline technique remains the same, the angle of needle insertion and the width of the interspinous space change. It is worth familiarising yourself with the difference in the shape of the lumbar, thoracic, and cervical vertebrae and the natural curves of the spinal column. You may consider a paramedian approach – see anaesthetic textbooks.

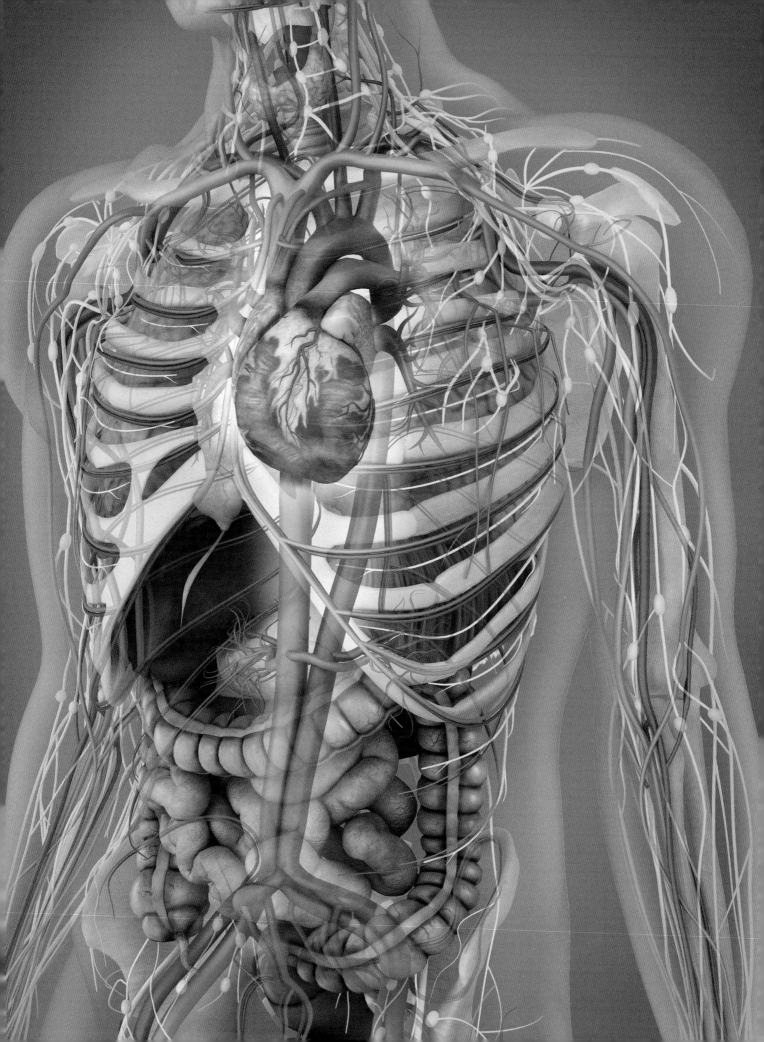

Procedure-related safety

Kirsty Cattle

Figure 40.1 List of 'Never Events', for which healthcare organisations have to set up mechanisms to prevent from ever occurring. Obtained from NHS Improvement.

Group	Never Event	Group	Never Event
Surgical	Wrong site surgery	Mental health	Failure to install functional collapsible shower or curtain rails
	Wrong implant/prosthesis	General	Falls from poorly restricted windows
	Retained foreign object post procedure		Chest or neck entrapment in bed rails
Medication	Mis-selection of a strong potassium solution		Transfusion or transplantation of ABO-incompatible blood components or organs
	Administration of medication by the wrong route		Misplaced naso- or oro-gastric tubes
	Overdose of insulin due to abbreviations or incorrect device		Scalding of patients
	Overdose of methotrexate for non-cancer treatment		Unintentional connection of a patient requiring oxygen to an air flowmeter
	Mis-selection of high strength midazolam during conscious sedation		Undetected oesophageal intubation

Figure 40.2 The Surgical Safety Checklist elements included in the WHO paper presenting significant improvement in patient outcomes after the introduction of the safer surgery checklist. Published by NEJM, 2009, volume 360, p491–9.

Table 1. Elements of the Surgical Safety Checklist.*

Sign in

Before induction of anesthesia, members of the team (at least the nurse and an anesthesia professional) orally confirm that:

- The patient has verified his or her identity, the surgical site and procedure, and consent
- The surgical site is marked or site marking is not applicable
- The pulse oximeter is on the patient and functioning
- All members of the team are aware of whether the patient has a known allergy
- The patient's airway and risk of aspiration have been evaluated and appropriate equipment and assistance are available
- If there is a risk of blood loss of at least 500 ml (or 7 ml/kg of body weight, in children), appropriate access and fluids are available

Time out

Before skin incision, the entire team (nurses, surgeons, anesthesia professionals, and any others participating in the care of the patient) orally:

- Confirms that all team members have been introduced by name and role
- Confirms the patient's identity, surgical site, and procedure
- Reviews the anticipated critical events
  - Surgeon reviews critical and unexpected steps, operative duration, and anticipated blood loss
  - Anesthesia staff review concerns specific to the patient
  - Nursing staff review confirmation of sterility, equipment availability, and other concerns
- Confirms that prophylactic antibiotics have been administered ≤60 min before incision is made or that antibiotics are not indicated
- Confirms that all essential imaging results for the correct patient are displayed in the operating room

Sign out

Before the patient leaves the operating room:

- Nurse reviews items aloud with the team
  - Name of the procedure as recorded
  - That the needle, sponge, and instrument counts are complete (or not applicable)
  - That the specimen (if any) is correctly labeled, including with the patient's name
  - Whether there are any issues with equipment to be addressed
- The surgeon, nurse, and anesthesia professional review aloud the key concerns for the recovery and care of the patient

* The checklist is based on the first edition of the WHO Guidelines for Safe Surgery.[15] For the complete checklist, see the Supplementary Appendix.

Applied Anatomy for Clinical Procedures at a Glance, First Edition. Jane Sturgess, Francesca Crawley, Ramez Kirollos, and Kirsty Cattle.
© 2021 John Wiley & Sons Ltd. Published 2021 by John Wiley & Sons Ltd.

The problem

- Estimated that 10% of hospital admissions suffer harm, half of which is considered preventable, resulting in long-term disability or death in 14% of cases. [1]
- Examples include hospital-acquired infections, falls, medication errors.
- Some medical errors are considered so severe in their consequences that these are termed 'Never Events' (Figure 40.1).
- Failures in care occur either because we do not (yet) know how to treat a condition (ignorance) or because we fail to apply known treatments (ineptitude).
- As medical knowledge increases in depth and breadth no one individual can hold all of it in their head, making ineptitude more likely.
- Medical staff do not turn up to work planning to harm patients.
- There are multiple organisational issues or human factors which lead or contribute to medical errors.

Definitions (as per the World Health Organisation)

- Error: the failure of a planned action to be completed as intended or use of a wrong, inappropriate, or incorrect plan to achieve an aim.
- Adverse event: an injury that was caused by medical management or complication instead of the underlying disease and that resulted in prolonged hospitalization or disability at the time of discharge from medical care, or both
- Near miss: an event that almost happened or an event that did happen but no one knows about. If the person involved in the near miss does not come forward, no one may ever know it occurred.
- Patient safety: the avoidance, prevention, and amelioration of adverse outcomes or injuries stemming from the processes of health care. These events include 'errors', 'deviations', and 'accidents'. Safety emerges from the interaction of the components of the system; it does not reside in a person, device, or department. Improving safety depends on learning how safety emerges from the interactions of the components. Patient safety is a subset of healthcare quality.

The response

- Training and education have been the traditional response to the problem of medical errors, with increasing specialisation and sub-specialisation, so that medical staff are more likely to be able to grasp the vast amount of increasing medical knowledge in their specific area of expertise.
- Learning from other complex organisations with safety at their core – for example, the airline industry
- Important to introduce a 'no blame culture'. Medical staff who make errors are more likely to report them or near misses, improving the chances of others learning from this mistake, if they do not fear punishment for making or admitting to a mistake.
- The World Health Organisation (WHO) ran a study implementing a checklist and 'stop points' in surgical care. This included three points at which the team stopped to ensure that certain key things had been done or checked (Figure 40.2).

The overall post-operative complication rate was significantly reduced after introduction of the checklist. [2]
- This has led to the universal use of checklists to improve surgical safety.
- National Safety Standards for Invasive Procedures (NatSSIPs) were introduced to bring the WHO surgical safety checklist approach to other invasive procedures, not necessarily carried out in an operating theatre.
- Local hospitals are encouraged to adapt NatSSIPs for their local setup and develop Local Safety Standards for Invasive Procedures (LocSSIPs).
- Safety standards address non-technical skills and human factors, not aimed at the technical performance of individual procedures.

Responsibilities for National Health Service (NHS) and staff

- The NHS has responded to safety concerns and recommendations from Sir Robert Francis QC by developing a national whistleblowing policy, encouraging staff to speak up and express concerns, as well as requiring NHS organisations to appoint whistleblowing guardians and investigate concerns raised by staff.
- The duties of a doctor, as laid out by the GMC in 'Good Medical Practice', include promoting and encouraging a culture which allows staff to raise concerns and requiring doctors to take action where patient safety, dignity or comfort are or may be compromised.

Top tips (from the World Health Organisation)

- Avoid reliance on memory
- Simplify
- Standardize
- Use constraints and forcing functions
- Use protocols and checklists wisely
- Improve information access
- Reduce handovers
- Increase feedback

References

1. Improving patient safety: Insights from American, Australian and British healthcare. Edited by Stuart Emslie, Kirstine Knox, Martin Pickstone. Published by ECRI Europe, 2002.
2. Haynes AB, Weiser TG, Berry WR, et al. A surgical safety checklist to reduce morbidity and mortality in a global population. *N Engl J Med* 2009; 360: 491–9.

Additional reading

1. Executive summary: In Institute of Medicine (US): To err is human: building a safer health system. Washington, National Academy Press 2000
2. Reason J. Human error: models and management. *BMJ* 2000; 320:786–90.
3. Leape LL. Error in medicine. *JAMA* 1994; 272:1851–7.
4. National Guardian's Office, www.cqc.org.uk/content/national-guardians-office
5. The duties of a doctor registered with the General Medical Council, www.gmc-uk.org/ethical-guidance/ethical-guidance-for-doctors/good-medical-practice/duties-of-a-doctor

Index

Note: Page numbers in *italic* refer to figures.

Applied Anatomy for Clinical Procedures at a Glance, First Edition. Jane Sturgess, Francesca Crawley, Ramez Kirollos, and Kirsty Cattle.
© 2021 John Wiley & Sons Ltd. Published 2021 by John Wiley & Sons Ltd.